Instructor's Manual and Testbank to Accompany

Timby/Smith's Introductory Medical-Surgical Nursing

EIGHTH EDITION

Joanne Carlson, MS, APRN, ANP-BC

Executive Director
Medical Career Development Centers, Inc.
Midvale, Utah

Visit the Lippincott Williams & Wilkins Website
http://www.lww.com

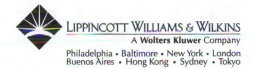

LIPPINCOTT WILLIAMS & WILKINS
A **Wolters Kluwer** Company

Philadelphia • Baltimore • New York • London
Buenos Aires • Hong Kong • Sydney • Tokyo

Ancillary Editor: Doris S. Wray
Compositor: LWW
Printer/Binder: Victor Graphics

ISBN: 0-7817-3700-1

Any procedure or practice described in this book should be applied by the health care practitioner under appropriate supervision in accordance with professional standards of care used with regard to the unique circumstances that apply in each practice situation. Care has been taken to confirm the accuracy of information presented and to describe generally accepted practices. However, the authors, editors, and publisher cannot accept any responsibility for errors or omissions or for any consequences from application of the information in this book and make no warranty, express or implied, with respect to the contents of the book.

Contents

UNIT 6
Caring for Clients With Respiratory Disorders

UNIT 7
Caring for Clients With Cardiovascular Disorders

UNIT 8
Caring for Clients With Hematopoietic and Lymphatic Disorders

UNIT 9
Caring for Clients With Immune Disorders

UNIT 10
Caring for Clients With Neurologic Disorders

UNIT 11
Caring for Clients With Sensory Disorders

UNIT 12
Caring for Clients With Gastrointestinal Disorders

UNIT 13
Caring for Clients With Endocrine Problems

UNIT 14
Sexual Structures and Reproductive Function

UNIT 15
Caring for Clients With Urinary and Renal Disorders

UNIT 16
Caring for Clients With Musculoskeletal Disorders

UNIT 17
Caring for Clients With Integumentary Disorders

Testbank and Testbank Answers (on Accompanying CD)

Guidelines for Evaluating Critical Thinking Exercises can be found on our Connection—LPN website: http://connection.lww.com

Concepts and Trends in Health Care

CHAPTER OVERVIEW

Chapter 1 introduces the student to the health profession and the impact on nursing. Health care delivery is defined as the range of services available to people who seek health and treatment for diseases. New trends in methods of payment for services are described.

KEY TERMS

Capitation	Illness
Client	Integrated delivery system
Critical pathways	Integrative medicine
Diagnosis-related groups	Managed care
Disease	organization
Health	Preferred provider
Health care delivery system	organization
Health care team	Primary care
Health maintenance	Prospective payment
Health maintenance	systems
organization	Secondary care
Health promotion	Tertiary care
Holism	Wellness

■ Case Studies

3. Mrs. Thibideau is a 75-year-old woman in reasonably good health who lives alone. Her deceased husband had worked in the city school system, and as part of his retirement benefits had insurance coverage from Blue Cross/Blue Shield for himself and his wife. After Mr. Thibideau died, the Blue Cross health insurance plan switched to a health maintenance organization (HMO) plan. Mrs. Thibideau was used to submitting her medical bills to the insurance company. Now she was required to select a new physician (her former physician was not a member of the HMO) and to pay a small co-payment fee for each office visit. If she wanted to see her rheumatologist, she had to have a referral from her primary care physician. She no longer needed to submit her medical bills to the insurance company; she only received statements regarding the bills. In many ways the new system was easier, but she missed her former physician and the freedom to see her specialist when she wanted to.

2. The post-surgical floor in an acute care hospital has a bed capacity of 40. With the increase in ambulatory or day surgery, the average census has dropped to 25. The surgical clients admitted to the unit are generally recovering from complex surgery and are in need of highly skilled care. Many of the clients are Medicare clients—the reimbursement is based on diagnostic-related groups (DRGs). In addition, a productivity study was recently done on this unit to determine what the staffing needs were on an average day. This study demonstrated that the registered nurse (RN) staff needed to be reduced by 4 full-time RNs and 2 full-time licensed practical nurses (LPNs). The study further recommended that 2 certified nurse's aides (CNAs) be added to the staff. The amount of supplies on the unit has been reduced to help control costs. Most items need to be ordered from Central Supply on an as-needed basis. A unit secretary works on two units so that he or she is on the unit for only one-half of the shift. Two of the aides have been crossed-trained to work as unit secretaries.

3. Janine is a 35-year-old woman, newly diagnosed with breast cancer. Her oncologist recommends a bilateral mastectomy with chemotherapy. Janine agrees to the mastectomy but wants to use alternative herbal therapy instead of chemotherapy. How might you respond to Janine's decision? What information should Janine have prior to making her final decision?

■ Internet Resources

Capitation: www.amso.com/capitation.html
Clinical Pathways:
   www.aapmr.org/memphys/pracguide/clinpath.htm
Managed Care: www.managedcaremag.com
Managed Care Nursing: www.aamcn.org

CHAPTER 2

Nursing in Various Settings

CHAPTER OVERVIEW

This chapter defines the concepts of nursing and models of nursing care. Two nursing theorists' viewpoints are shared, as is the American Nurses Association (ANA) definition. Numerous settings for nursing care are identified with the aspect of care they provide to clients.

KEY TERMS

Assisted living
Boarding homes
Case management
Case method
Congregate housing

Functional nursing
Home health care
Patient-focused care
Primary nursing
Team nursing

■ Case Study

1. Timothy is a 57-year-old single man with diabetes. After a recent fracture of his hip, he was hospitalized for 5 days while in traction. He no longer needs acute care and is being readied for discharge. He will continue to need intravenous infusion of antibiotics for 5 more days and will need daily insulin injections. He will not be weight bearing for 6 more weeks. What is the best setting, in terms of costs and quality of care, for him to complete his recuperation and rehabilitation?

■ Internet Resources

American Hospital Association: www.aha.org
Home Health Care: www.nahc.org/hhna
Hospice and Palliative Association: www.hpna.org
National Association for Home Care: www.nahc.org
Office Nurses: www.aaon.org

The Nursing Process

CHAPTER OVERVIEW

Chapter 3 introduces the student to the nursing process. The nursing process provides the framework for nursing care in all settings. Therefore, mastering the steps to the nursing process and learning critical thinking skills are essential to success in the nursing profession. The purpose of the nursing process is to provide a method for nurses to systematically plan and implement client care to achieve desired outcomes. It is a dynamic and continuous process. Nursing diagnoses are developed with the RN to identify and define actual or potential problems. The North American Nursing Diagnosis Association (NANDA) developed a classification system for client problems. These diagnoses can be used in all health settings. Actual diagnoses identify existing problems, whereas risk diagnoses identify potential problems. Possible problems indicate uncertainty, and collaborative problems denote complications with a physiologic origin. Wellness diagnoses begin with the stem "potential for enhanced," and syndrome diagnoses identify a diagnosis associated with a cluster of other diagnoses before self-actualization. Critical thinking is intentional, contemplative, and outcome-directed thinking used during the nursing process. Critical thinking skills can be developed by the student using purposeful, outcome-directed thinking, combined with the basic principles of the nursing process and scientific method. An inquiring mind is necessary to re-evaluate, revise, and strive for improvement.

KEY TERMS

Actual diagnosis	Interventions
Assessment	Nursing diagnosis
Client database	Nursing orders
Collaborative problems	Nursing process
Critical thinking	Planning
Documentation	Possible diagnosis
Evaluation	Risk diagnosis
Expected outcomes	Syndrome diagnosis
Implementation	Wellness diagnosis

■ Case Studies

1. Mrs. Williams, 59 years old, was admitted to the hospital with colon cancer. Surgery was planned for the following day, with a probable colostomy. The RN who admitted the client had to hurry through the admission assessment because she had to admit and administer medications to two other clients. She planned to have the evening nurse do the preoperative teaching. When Mrs. Williams returned from surgery, the RN caring for the client told Mrs. Williams that she arranged for the enterostomal therapist to see her to begin teaching her about her colostomy. Mrs. Williams was very upset with this and asked why she had not been asked about this. She has assisted her husband for 5 years in taking care of his colostomy and feels very comfortable with the procedures. Mrs. Williams was also concerned that her insurance plan would not cover consultation services.

2. It has been a busy day on the rehabilitation unit in a long-term care facility. Henry Jordan, RN, is with a transfer client from the hospital, in addition to managing the care for 10 other clients. He asks the LPN to collect the admission data so that he can follow up with some other client issues. The LPN notes that the new client has staples in a left hip incision: the client was in the hospital for 2 weeks after a total hip replacement because of postoperative complications that included pneumonia and thrombophlebitis. The client is 70 years old. When Henry quickly reviews the admission data, he notes that the client needs to concentrate on increasing her ambulation and becoming

independent with activities of daily living. Three days after the client's admission to the rehabilitation unit, the client's temperature is elevated, and there is evidence of a wound infection.

3. Lucy Devlin has been an RN for 12 years. For the last 6 years, she has worked as a charge nurse on a skilled care facility. She was recently helping a client plan for a transfer to an assisted living center. This client had a cerebral vascular accident with residual left-sided weakness. She can ambulate with a walker and is now able to meet most of her self-care needs, but she has some difficulty with meal preparation and housekeeping. This client tells Lucy that she is concerned about taking care of her finances.

Although Lucy is not sure whether the assisted living center has financial services available to its residents, she tells the client that she need not worry about that because all of her financial issues will be eliminated once she moves to the assisted living center. What would have been a better approach?

■ Internet Resources

Care Planning:
    http://dmoz.org/Health/Nursing/Care_Plans
Nursing Process:
    www.uri.edu/nursing/schmieding/orlando

Physical Assessment

CHAPTER OVERVIEW

Chapter 4 introduces the student to the assessment phase of the nursing process. Findings from the assessment will be used to establish a database from which to develop a plan of care. Methods to complete the assessment are the interview and physical examination. Physical examination is the collection of objective data. Physical examination may be accomplished by a systems approach or the head-to-toe method. The nurse should examine not only body structures but also the client's physical appearance, mood, mental status, behaviors, and ability to interact during the process. Assessment techniques include inspection, palpation, percussion, and auscultation. Physical assessment requires practice and should be provided in such a way as to maintain the client's privacy. The patient should be kept as covered and warm as possible during the process. General gerontologic considerations are included to assist the student when working with this population.

KEY TERMS

Auscultation
Chief complaint
Closed questions
Cultural history
Focus assessment
Functional assessment
Head-to-toe method
Inspection
Objective data
Open-ended questions
Palpation
Past health history
Percussion
Physical assessment
Psychosocial history
Signs
Subjective data
Symptoms
Systems method

■ Case Study

1. Mr. Granger is a 79-year-old Alzheimer's patient who is admitted to the floor with a suspected broken hip. What special needs might Mr. Granger have prior to beginning the interview and physical assessment? What nursing interventions can you perform to accommodate the physical examination process better?

■ Lippincott Williams & Wilkins Multimedia Resources

Assessment Throughout the Lifespan, video (1996)
Assessment of the Older Adult, video (1996)
Performing Head-to-Toe Assessment, video (2000)

■ Internet Resources

Physical Assessment:
    http://nursingabout.com/cs/assessmentskills
Physical Assessment:
    http://www.cp-tel.net/pamnorth/assess.htm

CHAPTER 5

Legal and Ethical Issues

CHAPTER OVERVIEW

Chapter 5 introduces the student to the legal and ethical issues inherent in the nursing profession. Sources of law are discussed in context to how they affect nursing practice.

KEY TERMS

Administrative law	Liability
Advance directives	Living will
Advocacy	Malpractice
Anecdotal record	Medical durable
Board of nursing	power of attorney
Civil law	Negligence
Common law	Nurse practice acts
Constitutional law	Rights
Criminal law	Risk management
Deontology	Statute of limitations
Duty	Statutory law
Ethics	Tort
Good Samaritan laws	Tort law
Incident report	Unintentional torts
Intentional tort	Utilitarianism
Laws	Values

■ Case Studies

1. An 89-year-old woman is admitted to an acute care unit with pneumonia. She has lived in the same home for the last 50 years and has lived alone for the past 10 years. Until the pneumonia developed, she had been independent, needing assistance only with transportation from a daughter who lives nearby. When admitted, she was having some difficulty breathing, particularly with exertion. She presented with a frequent unproductive cough. She was alert when admitted but had to be reminded occasionally where she was. As evening came, she was more confused. She could not remember where she was or why she was there. The nurse showed her how to use the call bell and instructed her to remain in bed. The client's daughter asked that the side rails be up so that her mother would be safe. The hospital policy required that the client or family member sign a permission form for side rails to be up. After the daughter left, the night nurse checked on the client and found her trying to climb over the side rails to get out of bed. The client told the nurse that she needed to check the stove.

2. A young man was in a motor vehicle accident and died as a result of his injuries. His liver was harvested for organ donation. Two possible recipients are identified. The first is a 16-year-old girl with a history of liver disease. She is a high-school sophomore who had previously been a strong academic student and a member of the student council. She also is an excellent violinist and played in the state youth orchestra. The second candidate is a 55-year-old gentleman with a history of liver disease. He owns a successful construction company, is married, with one child in college and another who is married with a new baby. If both match for the liver, the organ transplant team will need to decide who should receive the liver.

3. A mildly confused, elderly client, Mrs. S., has liver cancer but is expected to live at least several more months. She eats and drinks, but overall her intake is poor. Efforts to have her drink and eat more have failed, and consent to place a feeding tube is obtained from her power of attorney. The physician asks the nurse to assist while the feeding tube is placed. Mrs. S resists placement, and her hands must be restrained to get the feeding tube down. The restraints must be applied indefinitely to prevent her from dislodging the tube.

4. Mrs. Jepson, age 69, has been admitted to an Alzheimer's unit in a long-term care facility by her husband. She is combative and has a poor attention span. She recognizes her daughter but no other family members. She is unable to dress or bathe herself but is able to ambulate and feed herself. How can the nurse protect Mrs. Jepson's rights (see Patients' Bill of Rights) while maintaining her safety? What are the legal and ethical issues in this case study?

■ Lippincott Williams & Wilkins Multimedia Resources

Clinical and Legal Ethics of Wound Care, video (1998)

■ Internet Resources

Legal Nurse Consultants: www.aalnc.org
Nurse Attorneys: www.taana.org
Nursing Ethics:
www.bc.edu/bc_org/avp/son/ethics/ethicsmain.html
Nursing Ethics Network:
www.nursingethicsnetwork.org

CHAPTER 6

Leadership Roles and Management Functions

CHAPTER OVERVIEW

This chapter provides an overview of theory related to leadership and management in relationship to the nurse manager. Autocratic, democratic, and laissez-faire leadership methods are defined. The role of licensed practical nurse (LPN) as a manger of patient care is explained in terms of responsibility and accountability. The LPN learns how to delegate and supervise ancillary personnel appropriately. Different methods of time management are discussed.

KEY TERMS

Accountability
Advocacy
Autocratic leadership
Collaboration
Delegation
Democratic leadership
Laissez-faire leadership

Leadership
Management
Power
Resource management
Responsibility
Supervision
Time management

■Case Studies

1. No one wants to take care of Mr. Beesley because he treats the unlicensed assistive personnel (UAPs) rudely, and his behavior is sexually inappropriate.

   - Identify positive and creative approaches to problem solving.
   - Which type of leadership style would be best used in this situation?
   - What is the best use of resources to resolve this problem?

2. During the past 2 months, there have been many complaints about a nursing assistant who has been employed at the facility for 15 years. She is difficult, bossy, and lazy.

   - What type of power does the LPN manager have?
   - What would be the best approach toward the UAP?
   - How can the LPN manager best handle the concerns of the other personnel?

■Internet Resources

National Federation of Licensed Practical/ Vocational Nurses: www.nflpn.org

CHAPTER 7

Biopsychosocial Aspects of Caring for Young Adults

CHAPTER OVERVIEW

Young adults may be described as Generation X and Y. Generation Y are individuals who graduated from college in 1998. Generation X was the group prior to Y. This age group is most likely to experience acute illness and trauma, with small numbers experiencing chronic diseases. Pregnancy can cause many unique physical changes. In addition to uterine and breast enlargement, changes occur in the circulatory system and skin and may occur in the thyroid gland. Tattoos and body piercing have become a growing trend in this age group. Both of these practices have brought new challenges in health care delivery.

KEY TERMS

Adolescent moratorium	Industry
Androgyny	Inferiority
Autonomy	Initiative
Blended family	Intimacy
Development	Isolation
Developmental stage	Mistrust
Developmental tasks	Nuclear family
Domestic violence	Personal protection order
Doubt	Psychosocial stages
Ego identity	Rape
Extended family	Role confusion
Gender role	Shame
Generation X	Single-parent family
Generation Y	Temporary restraining
Growth	order
Guilt	Traditional family
	Trust

■ Case Study

1. Stephanie is a 22-year-old grocery store clerk. She presents in the emergency department (ED) with a broken ulna. She has bruises in different stages of healing on her back, thigh, and abdomen. Stephanie is 5 months pregnant. She claims to have lost her balance and fallen down the stairs at home. Stephanie's significant other is waiting in the waiting area. Stephanie has a one-pack-a-day cigarette habit and drinks beer and wine occasionally. In what developmental stage should Stephanie be? If you suspect domestic violence, how would you approach this with Stephanie? What health problems can you identify for Stephanie? Prioritize the nursing diagnoses, and identify how you would approach each one.

■ Lippincott Williams & Wilkins Multimedia Resources

Assessment Throughout the Lifespan, video (1996)

Lippincott's Clinical Assessment Skills Series, video (1997)

■ Internet Resources

Ambulatory Care: www.aaacn.inurse.com

CHAPTER 8

Biopsychosocial Aspects of Caring for Middle-Aged Adults

CHAPTER OVERVIEW

Middle age, from 35 to 65 years, is characterized as the established years. During this period, the individual has a chance to actualize the earlier struggles to establish a home and career. Middle-aged adults have the opportunity to analyze their assets and channel their energies into accomplishing life goals that are unfulfilled.

KEY TERMS

Basal metabolic rate (BMR)
Generativity
Keratotic lesion
Menopause
Mid-life crisis
Osteoporosis
Presbycusis
Presbyopia
Sandwich generation
Stagnation

■ Case Studies

1. A 50-year-old is admitted to the emergency room with complaints of severe substernal chest pain. The emergency room staff take measures to stabilize his condition and then transfer him to the coronary intensive care unit. After 24 hours, he remains in stable condition but is anxious and depressed. He is a successful owner of a dry cleaning business. He and his wife have been married for 25 years. Their two children have graduated from college and are doing well in their jobs. This client regrets that his business often prevented him from spending more time with his family, and he was not always able to be involved in community activities.

2. A home health nurse makes a visit to an elderly client to assess her ability to perform activities of daily living. This client lives with her 48-year-old daughter. She has her own bedroom and bathroom and a small kitchenette. She frequently eats meals with her daughter and family but is able to fix simple meals without too much difficulty. After assessing the client, the nurse meets with the daughter. The daughter states that lately her mother is more forgetful and that she has had to disconnect the stove in the kitchenette. Her mother is also weaker than usual and has difficulty bathing and dressing. The daughter works as a management consultant and travels frequently. The daughter's husband is home most evenings, but he often brings work home. Their 19-year-old daughter is attending the local community college, working on a degree in computer science. The client's daughter worries that her mother is alone too much and is unable to care for herself as well as she used to. She is also concerned that her husband and daughter are required to provide more assistance to the client than they want or have time to do.

■ Lippincott Williams & Wilkins Multimedia Resources

Assessment Throughout the Lifespan, video (1996)
Lippincott's Clinical Assessment Skills Series, video (1997)
Performing Head to Toe Assessment, video (2000)
Safe Back Workout, video (1998)
Visual Guide to Physical Assessment, video (1995)

■ Internet Resources

Middle-age issues: http:ohioline.osu.edu/hyg-fact/5000/5221.html

CHAPTER 9

Biopsychosocial Aspects of Caring for Older Adults

CHAPTER OVERVIEW

Older adults play a vital role in society, the home, the workplace, and the community. They offer others with less maturity the wisdom of life experiences. Health care workers play an important role in helping older adults maintain their independence, health, and productivity. Older adults struggle with the developmental task for ego integrity versus stagnation. Elders spend much time on life review and often plan their own burials and disposition of their belongings. The nurse plays an important role in supporting the gradual decline of the client.

KEY TERMS

Ageism	Kyphosis
Antioxidants	Life review
Autophagocytosis	Pet therapy
Ego integrity	Reality orientation
Elder abuse	Reminiscence therapy
Free radicals	Senescence
Gerontology	Validation therapy

■ Case Studies

1. An 85-year-old woman is transferred from an acute care hospital to a rehabilitation center after a total hip replacement. Her recovery at the hospital was complicated by pneumonia, which required 7 days of intravenous antibiotics. She plans to return to her home, which is in the same town as the rehabilitation center. This client has lived in this home for the past 15 years. Her husband passed away 5 years ago. One of her sons lives in the next town. The house is a one-floor ranch style home. One entrance is handicapped accessible; her husband had needed a wheelchair prior to his death. The client tells the nurse that she will only need to be at the center until she is independent. She states that she has no intention of remaining in a "home" for the elderly.

2. Mr. K. is a 90-year-old gentleman who recently moved into a long-term care facility. He had been living by himself in an apartment, but his family persuaded him to move. They had noted that his memory was not good, especially regarding time and place. He was also confused about when to take his medications, and they were afraid that he would harm himself by making a mistake. Mr. K. needs to be reminded about where he is; much of the time he believes that he is in his apartment.

■ Lippincott Williams & Wilkins Multimedia Resources

Assessment Throughout the Lifespan, video (1996)
Lippincott's Clinical Assessment Skills Series, video (1997)
Performing Head to Toe Assessment, video (2000)
Visual Guide to Physical Assessment, video (1995)

■ Internet Resources

American Association of Retired Persons:
   www.aarp.org/
Geriatric Discussion Group:
   www.santel.lu/SANTEL/geriatrics/gerinet.html

CHAPTER 10

Nurse-Client Relationships

CHAPTER OVERVIEW

Chapter 10 introduces the student to the concept of the nurse-client relationship. Therapeutic communication, empathetic listening, sharing information, and providing client education are techniques used to establish and promote this alliance.

KEY TERMS

Affective learner	Learning style
Affective touch	Listening
Caregiver	Motivation
Cognitive learner	Nonverbal communication
Collaborator	Nurse-client relationship
Comfort zone	Paralanguage
Delegator	Personal space
Educator	Proxemics
Empathy	Psychomotor learner
Formal teaching	Public space
Hearing	Social space
Informal teaching	Task-oriented touch
Intimate space	Teaching plan
Introductory phase	Terminating phase
Kinesics	Therapeutic communication
Learning capacity	Verbal communication
Learning needs	Working phase
Learning readiness	

■ Case Studies

1. The nurse is teaching her client how to change his ileostomy bag. The client keeps his eyes focused on the nurse while she is changing the ileostomy pouch. He does not respond in any way to what she is saying. The nurse finally says, "You have told me and your physician that it will not be a problem to manage your ileostomy, and yet you will not even look at what I am doing." The client shouts, "I hate this thing—I can't believe I am stuck with this thing for the rest of my life!"

2. Mrs. J. tells her nurse, "I am really scared about my surgery tomorrow. I am afraid that I will not do well." The nurse tells her, "You don't have a thing to worry about. You have an excellent doctor and you will be in good hands."

   Mrs. J. tells her nurse, "I am really scared about my surgery tomorrow. I am afraid that I will not do well." The nurse waits for a while, maintaining eye contact with the client. Mrs. J then tells the nurse that her sister died during surgery 2 years ago. The nurse says, "You must be very frightened."

3. The nurse is preparing to teach several clients about their upcoming surgery. Keeping in mind that there are various learning styles, the nurse plans several approaches for the teaching:

   Cognitive—handouts listing the postoperative expectations

   Affective—discussion of usual preoperative concerns and methods to alleviate anxiety

   Psychomotor—a demonstration and return demonstration of postoperative exercises and pulmonary exercises

4. A newly graduated LPN prepares to enter Ted Ferris's room for the first time. Ted is a 65-year-old man admitted with the diagnoses of hypertension. What are the steps to beginning the nurse-client relationship? How can the LPN facilitate each phase? What should the LPN do if the client is not ready to terminate the relationship after the health problem has been resolved?

■ Lippincott Williams & Wilkins Multimedia Resources

Communication Skills, CD-ROM (1998)

CHAPTER 11

Caring for Culturally Diverse Clients

CHAPTER OVERVIEW

People vary in many ways, including age, gender, country of origin, language, education, and religion. These differences impact their belief system and health practices. Nurses need to be aware of a multitude of cultural concepts and develop the ability to communicate with many cultures. A cultural assessment assists the nurse in providing care unique to the individual. Transcultural nursing is considered a specialty in nursing. Developing cultural competence assists the nurse in providing care outside his or her own cultural context.

KEY TERMS

Cultural competence

Culture

Ethnicity

Ethnocentrism

Generalization

Health beliefs

Health practices

Minority

Race

Stereotyping

Subculture

Transcultural nursing

■ Case Studies

1. A home health nurse has been assigned to admit a new client to the agency. From the intake information and the transfer report from the hospital, the nurse learns that the client is 62 years old. She had a total abdominal hysterectomy 8 days ago and developed a wound infection while in the hospital. The wound requires daily wet to dry dressing changes. The client lives with her 85-year-old mother in an apartment. The client is originally from Vietnam and has been in this country for 12 years. She is separated from her husband. Two grown children live nearby.

2. The nurse on a surgical floor is assigned to care for a client who had a below-the-knee amputation 3 days ago. She is an insulin-dependent diabetic. The client is from India. The client's two daughters, mother, sister, brother, brother's wife, and brother's two children appear and bring their own food to eat with the client. The client refuses the hospital food but eats what her family brings her. The nurse is uncertain what the food is and if it is appropriate for the client's 1800-calorie ADA diet.

3. An African-American client made an appointment to see her physician because she had been feeling dizzy, had frequent headaches, and generally did not feel well. The nurse noted that the client was tall and was at least 50 lb overweight. The client's blood pressure was 200/110. The nurse knew that African-Americans were prone to hypertension and obesity. Calling the client by her first name, she asked if anyone had talked to her about a weight-reduction program, including diet and exercise regimens. When the client did not respond, the nurse simply said that the physician would be with her in a few minutes.

■ Lippincott Williams & Wilkins Multimedia Resources

Cultural Diversity in Healthcare, video (1994)

■ Internet Resources

Transcultural Nursing Basic Concepts and Case Studies: www.culturediversity.org

Transcultural Nursing Healthcare: www.fons.org/networks/tchnha/

Transcultural Nursing Organization: www.tcnhs.org

CHAPTER 12

Interaction of Body and Mind

CHAPTER OVERVIEW

Chapter 12 introduces the student to the body and mind connection. Psychobiology, psychoneurology, and pyschoimmunology are presented as new fields of science that affect health care. Assessment and diagnosis of mental disorders is based upon specific criteria listed in the *Diagnostic and Statistical Manual of Mental Disorders* (DSM-IV-TR). Assessment should include a comprehensive personal and family medical history, mental status examination, psychological testing, and laboratory and diagnostic testing.

KEY TERMS

Acupuncture
Alternative medical systems
Alternative therapy
Apitherapy
Aromatherapy
Neuropeptides
Ayurvedic medicine
Biofeedback
Biologic-based therapies
Body-based therapies
Brain mapping
Chinese medicine
Chiropractic
Complementary therapy
Coping mechanisms
Distress
Electromagnetic therapy
Energy therapies
Eustress
General adaptation
  syndrome
Hardiness
Herbal therapy
Humor
Hypnosis
Imagery
Immunopeptides

Limbic system
Massage therapy
Mental status
  examination
Mind-body
  interventions
Neurotransmitters
Placebo
Placebo effect
Psyche
Psychobiologic
  disorders
Psychobiology
Psychoneuroendocrinology
Psychoneuroimmunology
Psychosomatic diseases
Receptor
Reflexology
Reiki
Shiatsu
Soma
Spiritual healing
Stress
Stress management
Tai chi
Yoga

■ Case Study

1. Timothy is a 24-year male client. He recently married his high school sweetheart and bought a new home. He was working a construction job but got laid off due to the poor economy. He had already purchased a new car but still has a large loan to pay. His wife was working but recently took a medical leave of absence due to a high-risk pregnancy. What score do you think Timothy will get on the Social Readjustment Rating Scale? What is his risk for developing an illness related to stress? What signs and symptoms would you expect Timothy to exhibit?

■ Lippincott Williams & Wilkins Multimedia Resources

Psychiatric Nursing Made Incredibly Easy! CD-ROM (2000)
Psychosocial Nursing Assessment, video (1992)

■ Internet Resources

Mental Health: www.mentalhealth.com
Neuroscience Nursing: www.aann.org
Psychiatric Nursing: www.apna.org

CHAPTER 13

Caring for Clients With Somatoform Disorders

CHAPTER OVERVIEW

Clients with somatoform disorders have no physiologic basis for their physical symptoms. They often go from doctor to doctor seeking relief from their symptoms. Somatoform disorders are conditions that result from somatization. The psychological origin of the client with somatoform disorders is unknown, and the client believes that the physical symptoms are real.

KEY TERMS

Body dysmorphic disorder
Conversion disorder
Factitious disorders
Histrionic
Hypochondriasis
Insight-oriented therapy
La belle indifference

Malingering
Muchausen's syndrome
Muchausen's syndrome
 by proxy
Somatic pain disorder
Somatization
Somatoform disorders

■ Case Studies

1. Mrs. N. presents with complaints of severe abdominal pain, cramping, and intermittent spasms in her bowels. Last week she went to a clinic with complaints of right hip pain that was so bad she had difficulty ambulating. She tells the nurse that she has seen different doctors in the past 2 months for various complaints, including shortness of breath, head and neck pain that kept her awake, and heart palpitations.

2. Mr. O. has been hospitalized for chronic complaints of pain in his back, arms, and shoulders. The physical examination and subsequent tests are negative. Mr. O.'s wife of 20 years recently served him with divorce papers and was granted custody of their two teenage children. The physical examination determines that the client has a somatoform disorder. The client is transferred to a psychiatric unit. The treatment plan includes the use of insight-oriented therapy.

■ Lippincott Williams & Wilkins Multimedia Resources

Psychosocial Nursing Assessment, video (1992)

■ Internet Resources

Alliance for Psychosocial Nursing:
 www.psychnurse.org
Issues in Mental Health Nursing:
 www.tandf.co.uk/journals/tf/01612840.html
Online Dictionary of Mental Health:
 www.human-nature.com/odmh/psnursing.html

Caring for Clients With Anxiety Disorders

CHAPTER OVERVIEW

Chapter 14 explores anxiety and fear and discusses how to intervene for an anxious client. It also explores anxiety disorders and nursing care of those who have them. Typically, clients with anxiety disorders will present with physical signs and symptoms rather than complaints of anxiety. Physical symptoms of increased blood pressure and tachycardia are common. Diagnosis of most anxiety disorders is based upon symptomatology and client history. Interventions for the anxious client include being available and attentive, maintaining contact, avoiding interrupting, helping problem-solve, and ensuring safety. Clients need a lot of education regarding their medical, drug, and dietary regimens to manage anxiety symptoms.

KEY TERMS

Anxiety	Cognitive therapy
Anxiety disorders	Desensitization
Behavioral therapy	Fear

■ Case Study

1. Mrs. Johnson is admitted to the surgical unit for a bilateral mastectomy secondary to breast cancer. As you try to do the preoperative teaching, Mrs. Johnson fidgets, avoids eye contact, and generally is inattentive. What might be the cause of her inattentiveness? How can you establish rapport with Mrs. Johnson and accomplish the preoperative teaching?

■ Lippincott Williams & Wilkins Multimedia Resources

Psychiatric Nursing Made Incredibly Easy!, CD-ROM (2000)
Psychosocial Nursing Assessment, video (1992)

■ Internet Resources

American Psychiatric Association: www.psych.org
Anxiety:
www.nimh.nih.gov/anxiety/anxietymenu.cfm

Caring for Clients With Mood Disorders

CHAPTER OVERVIEW

Chapter 15 explores a variety of mood disorders. Clients with mood disorders experience extreme and persistent changes in affect that interfere with social relationships. Transient depression, or reactive depression, is a normal reaction to loss or disappointment. Typically, it is self-limiting and short in nature. Major or unipolar depression is a sad feeling with no obvious relationship to situation events. Moods are most likely generated in the limbic system. Mood disorders tend to be related to genetics, dysregulation or neurotransmitters, and neuroendocrine imbalances. Drug and psychotherapy are the most commonly used treatments for depression. A major role for nurses is to assist with activities of daily living as depressed clients often lack the energy or desire to participate in their own care.

KEY TERMS

Affect	Mood
Bipolar disorder	Mood disorders
Delusions	Norepinephrine
Dexamethasone (cortisol)	Photoperiods
suppression test	Phototherapy
Dopamine	Psychomotor agitation
Electroconvulsive therapy	Psychomotor retardation
Euthymic	Psychotherapy
Gamma aminobutyric acid	Psychotic depression
Hallucinations	Reactive (secondary)
Hypertensive crisis	depression
Hypothesis	Reuptake
Major (unipolar)	Seasonal affective
depression	disorder
Mania	SerotoninMonoamine
Melatonin	Serotonin syndrome

■ Case Studies

1. A nurse has been assigned to two clients. The first client, Mr. K., has been very morose for several days. He tells the nurse that he has nothing to live for, that there is no hope. The other client, Mr. D., has expressed that he wants to kill himself but does not have a gun to carry it out. The nurse recognizes that a plan of care must be developed to meet these clients' needs.

2. Ms. L. has been diagnosed with bipolar disease. She is in an acute care psychiatric setting. The nurse assesses that the client is in a manic episode because she is talking rapidly and loudly to anyone who will listen. Earlier, she had been very angry with the nurse who tried to calm her. She has not been able to sleep since admission, but instead spends the nights pacing the halls and barging into the other client's rooms. She occasionally kicks at furniture and doors as she moves rapidly down the hall. The nurse meets with the rest of the staff to plan for the safety needs of this client.

3. Ms. L's parents have a meeting with the staff to begin planning for her discharge and outpatient care. Ms. L's mother describes the strain that they have experienced in the past few months, knowing that there was something very wrong with their daughter. They never knew what mood she would be in. At times she was withdrawn and sad, unable to interact in any way. At other times her behavior was erratic and unpredictable. One of them always stayed up with her when she could not sleep because they were afraid that she would get hurt. The mother states that she does not know if she can cope any longer with her daughter's mental illness.

4. Jennifer is a 16-year-old client admitted to the locked mental health ward with the medical diagnosis major depression. Jennifer has attempted suicide by swallowing a bottle of Tylenol. Describe the steps involved in establishing suicide precautions for Jennifer.

■ Lippincott Williams & Wilkins Multimedia Resources

Psychiatric Nursing Made Incredibly Easy, CD-ROM (2000)
Psychosocial Nursing Assessment, video (1992)

■ Internet Resources

American Psychiatric Association: www.psych.org
Support Group: www.mdsg.org

CHAPTER 16

Caring for Clients With Eating Disorders

CHAPTER OVERVIEW

Eating disorders affect 500,000 people in the United States. Often the disorders are kept secret and not identified until serious health consequences occur. Neurotransmitters and neurohormones influence eating by binding with receptors in the appetite center of the hypothalamus. Medical management involves weight reduction, psychotherapy, and self-help support groups. SSRIs may be used to promote weight loss. Nursing interventions should include referral to a dietician, with a food plan that includes three meals and three snacks per day.

KEY TERMS

Anorexia nervosa	Leptin
Binge-eating disorder	Melanin-concentrating
Body mass index	hormone
Bulimarexia	Normal eating
Bulimia nervosa	Orexin A
Compulsive overeating	Orexin
Eating disorders	Purge
Endocannabinoids	Satiety
Food binges	Water loading
Lanugo	

■ Case Study

1. Cindy is a 15-year-old high school student who wants to go away to camp this summer. Cindy has been struggling with anorexia nervosa for 3 years. She is 5 ft 7 in tall and usually maintains her weight at 101 lb. Identify a goal weight for Cindy and a plan for her to maintain her weight while away at camp.

■ Lippincott Williams & Wilkins Multimedia Resources

Psychiatric Nursing Made Incredibly Easy!, CD-ROM (2000)
Psychosocial Nursing Assessment, video (1992)

■ Internet Resources

Anorexia: www.anred.com
Eating Disorders: www.nationaleatingdisorders.org

Caring for Chemically Dependent Clients

CHAPTER OVERVIEW

Chapter 17 discusses clients with substance abuse and chemical dependency problems. These are serious public health and social problems. These problems contribute significantly to morbidity and mortality. The primary abuse is with drugs that produce mind-altering and mood-altering effects. Withdrawal occurs when the drugs are reduced or stopped and physical symptoms and cravings occur. Alcoholism is a chronic, progressive, multisystem disease characterized by an inability to control the consumption of alcohol. It is generally accepted that there may be a genetic component to this disease. Treatment may include chemical detoxification and a plan that includes abstinence, counseling, and support groups. Twelve-step programs are a method to assist individuals to admit their disease and find new ways to cope with daily stressors. Nursing management for a client with an addiction includes assessing levels of intoxication, obtaining a health history of drug and alcohol abuse using the CAGE Screening test, and implementing protocols for detoxification. Maintaining the client's safety during the process of detoxification is paramount.

KEY TERMS

Alcoholism	Methadone
Aversion therapy	maintenance therapy
Blackouts	Opiate dependence
Chemical dependence	Polydrug abuse
Cross-tolerance	Relapse
Detoxification	Rule of One Hundreds
Employee or peer	Substance abuse
assistance programs	Tolerance
Environmental tobacco smoke	Withdrawal
Impaired nurse	

■ Case Studies

1. A client is admitted to a detoxification unit with a history of cocaine and alcohol abuse. He began having occasional drinks as a teenager and then experimented with cocaine while he was in college. His intake of both substances continued to increase. He tells the intake nurse that he needed the cocaine to feel good, but found that the alcohol helped him to sleep. This client is now 29 years old and has been unable to hold a job for 2 years. Last week he was involved in a motor vehicle accident while driving under the influence. Although no one was hurt, he was convicted of driving under the influence. He has been ordered by the court to undergo drug and alcohol detoxification and rehabilitation.

2. A client is admitted to a medical unit with acute respiratory symptoms related to chronic bronchitis. The client states that he has smoked two packs of cigarettes for the the past 20 years. He knows that he needs to quit smoking, but previous attempts have failed. He asks the nurse for suggestions to help him to quit smoking.

3. Sylvia is a 35-year old LPN working on a 35-bed medical-surgical unit. You have noticed that she seems forgetful, she claims to have dropped ampules of narcotics on more than one occasion, and the narcotic count is always off when Sylvia works. You begin to suspect Sylvia is abusing narcotics. What is your next step? What is your obligation? With whom will you discuss your concerns? What does your state law require? Are employee assistance programs available for professionals in your state?

■ Internet Resources

Habits: www.cts.com/crash/habtsmrt
International Nurses Society on Addictions:
  www.insta.org
National Clearinghouse for Alcohol & Drug
  Information (NCADI): www.health.org
Prevention:
  www.drugs.indiana.edu/druginfo/home.html
Web of Addictions: www.well.com/user/woa

CHAPTER 18

Caring for Clients With Dementia and Thought Disorders

CHAPTER OVERVIEW

Delirium is a sudden, transient state of confusion. Clients appear disoriented as to date, time, and/or location. Judgment is impaired, and clients may become suspicious or frightened. Delirium can result from high fever, head trauma, drug or alcohol intoxication or withdrawal, metabolic disorders, or inflammatory processes. Delirium is often reversed when the cause is resolved. Dementia is a condition in which memory and other mental functions decline. Alzheimer's disease is a leading example of dementia. Cerebrovascular disorders and Parkinson's disease can also cause dementia. Dementia is more likely to be a gradual process with little chance of reversibility. Nursing management is geared towards helping the client and the caregiver maintain the highest level of functioning and quality of life while ensuring safety.

KEY TERMS

Acalculia	Durable power of attorney
Acetylcholine	Extrapyramidal symptoms
Agnosia	Guardianship
Agraphia	Hallucinations
Alexia	Homocysteine
Alzheimer's disease	Incompetent
Aphasia	Mentation
Apraxia	Negative symptoms
Ataxia	Neuritic plaques
Beta amyloid	Neurofibrillary tangles
Cognitive functions	Positive symptoms
Conservatorship	Prions
Delirium	Respite care
Delusions	Restraint alternatives
Dementia	Schizophrenia
Depot injections	Voice dismissal

■ Case Study

1. Mr. Potter, a 72-year-old Alzheimer's client, is experiencing increasing periods of disorientation, agitation, and loss of the ability to communicate. His wife of 50 years says he wanders, and she has lost him twice in the grocery store this week. After performing an assessment, the nurse rates his deterioration as 6, middle dementia, on the Global Deterioration Scale. Develop a plan of care for Mr. Potter. What are his priority needs? How will you approach Mrs. Potter about possible admission of Mr. Potter to a long-term care facility?

■ Lippincott Williams & Wilkins Multimedia Resources

Clinical Simulations: Mental Health Nursing, CD-ROM (2000)
Neuroscience Nursing Videos, video (1995)

CHAPTER 19

Caring for Clients With Infectious Disorders

CHAPTER OVERVIEW

Infectious disorders are caused by microorganisms that invade the body. These organisms either cause the body's immune system to eliminate them, reside in the body without causing disease, or cause an infection or infectious disease. Infection occurs if the reservoir is suitable; it goes through a portal of exit by a mode of transmission, to a portal of entry, to a susceptible host, and then encounters the body's defense mechanisms. Infections may be localized or generalized and can be diagnosed through a variety of diagnostic tests. Medical management may include drug therapy, débridement of a wound, or wound irrigations. Nursing management includes nursing assessment, preparation for diagnostic tests, and specimen collection. The most important nursing care includes thorough handwashing with soap. The nurse must also follow standard precautions to avoid transmission of infectious microorganisms and nosocomial infections. Nursing management includes client and family teaching related to infection prevention, nutrition, pharmacology, and gerontologic considerations, as well as prevention of needle stick injuries.

KEY TERMS

Bacteremia
Carrier
Community-acquired
    infections
Culture
Fomites
Host
Infectious process cycle
Leukocytosis
Means of transmission
Microorganisms
Multi-drug resistance
Nonpathogens
Noscomial infections
Opportunistic infections

Pathogens
Phagocytosis
Portal of entry
Portal of exit
Prion
Reservoir
Sensitivity
Sepsis
Septicemia
Superinfections
Susceptibility
Transmission-based
    precautions
Virulence

■ Case Studies

1. Janet Markam enters the elevator in her office building early on a wintry morning to travel to her 11th-floor office. Because she is running a few minutes late, Janet decides to squeeze onto the elevator. At the front of the elevator, a gentleman sneezes and then begins to cough. Janet leaves the elevator on the 11th floor and enters her office. She hasn't been sleeping or eating well lately because she has been visiting her 75-year-old mother who is in the hospital's rehabilitation unit recovering from a fractured hip. A few days later, Janet awakens with rhinitis, a mild fever, and malaise.

2. Mary Jones, RN, is employed as a staff nurse on a busy surgical unit of a local hospital. When Mary arrives for work today, she learns that two nurses are absent because of the flu. This means that Mary and her coworkers are each assigned eight clients. Mary's assignment involves two clients who are scheduled for surgery and will be receiving preoperative intramuscular medications. The remaining six clients are recovering from surgical procedures; all have surgical sounds, and one is scheduled to be discharged. Mary's first two tasks are administration of meperidine 50 mg intramuscularly to Mr. Johnson for pain, and abdominal wound irrigation for Mrs. Treman, who is still receiving intravenous therapy.

3. Sally Rowen, RN, is caring for Mr. Lucas, a 75-year-old client who is on bed rest and is recovering from abdominal surgery. Mr. Lucas in on his fourth postoperative day when Sally assesses his lungs and hears mild crackles, which

she reports to Mr. Lucas' physician. After sending a sputum culture to the lab, Mr. Lucas' physician orders intravenous antibiotic therapy to treat potential pneumonia.

■ Internet Resources

Centers for Disease Control and Prevention:
  www.cdc.gov
Infection Control Nurses Association:
  www.icna.co.uk
Infection Control Today:
  www.infectioncontroltoday.com

CHAPTER 20

Caring for Clients With Cancer

CHAPTER OVERVIEW

The characteristics of cancer include abnormal, unrestricted cell proliferation. New growths of abnormal cells are called neoplasms or tumors, which can metastasize to other body tissues. Factors that cause cancer are termed carcinogens and can include chemicals, environmental agents, dietary issues, viruses, hormones, and familial or genetic influences. Research has increased public awareness of cancer-causing agents and risk factors. Specialized tests can aid in the diagnosis of cancer. Tumors are staged according to the ways they grow and the particular cell types. The TNM and other classification systems of tumors are used to determine specific treatments. The three major treatments of cancer include surgical removal of the tumor(s), chemotherapy, and radiation. Other therapies include bone marrow transplantation, biotherapies, gene therapy, and other alternative therapies. Adverse effects of treatment include hair loss, nausea and vomiting, suppression of immune systems, stomatitis, and fibrosis. The use of the nursing process provides a framework for implementation and evaluation of nursing care.

KEY TERMS

Alopecia	Leukopenia
Antineoplastic	Malignant
Apheresis	Metastasis
Benign	Myelosuppression
Brachytherapy	Neoplasms
Cancer	Neutropenia
Carcinogens	Oncology nursing
Chemotherapy	Radiation therapy
Engraftment	Stomatitis
Extravasation	Thrombocytopenia
Gene therapy	Vesicants
Immunotherapy	

■ Case Studies

1. Mrs. Jonkins, age 67, has been told that she will be hospitalized and treated with internal radiation therapy for endometrial cancer. Her daughter is with her during the admission process. After taking a nursing history, Carol Evans, RN, determines that Mrs. Jonkins' knowledge of the treatment regimen is very limited. Carol formulates a teaching plan for Mrs. Jonkins and her daughter.

2. Jonathan Pillman, age 12, is admitted to the hospital for an allogeneic bone marrow transplantation following a diagnosis of leukemia. Jonathan's parents are with him at the time of admission. Jack Sampson, RN, is assigned to admit Jonathan to the unit. During the nursing history, Jack determines that Jonathan understands very little about the scheduled procedure. Jack decides to develop a teaching plan for Jonathan and his parents.

■ Lippincott Williams & Wilkins Multimedia Resources

Cancer: Principles of Oncology, CD-ROM (2000)

■ Internet Resources

Cancer Guide: http://www.cancerguide.org
American Cancer Society: www.cancer.org
Cancer Prevention: www.ctrc.saci.org

Caring for Clients With Pain

CHAPTER OVERVIEW

Chapter 21 discusses clients experiencing pain. Pain is a personal experience with an unpleasant sensation usually associated with disease or injury. This chapter discusses ways in which the nurse can assist clients relieve or adapt to pain.

KEY TERMS

Acute pain	Pain perception
Addiction	Pain threshold
Adjuvant drugs	Pain tolerance
Analgesic	Pattern theory
Chronic pain	Perception
Endogenous opiates	Physical dependence
Equianalgesic dose	Referred pain
Gate-closing mechanisms	Somatic pain
Gate control theory	Specificity theory
Intractable pain	Substance P
Modulation	Tolerance
Neuropathic pain	Transduction
Nociceptive pain	Transmission
Nociceptors	Visceral pain
Pain	Withdrawal
Pain management	symptoms

■ Case Studies

1. Mr. Carson, a 67-year-old gentleman, has just been admitted to the orthopedic unit on a stretcher from the emergency room. He is being admitted to the unit after falling from a ladder and fracturing his right foot and hip. Surgery is scheduled in 1 hour. He is conscious but has a reddened face with his eyes shut. He states that he is in acute pain. He says to the nurse, "Can't you just give me something to knock me out?"

2. Marsha Stevens, RN, is employed on a busy orthopedic unit. She is assigned to care for Mrs. Bonhart, a 55-year-old client who has just returned from surgery after fracturing her wrist from falling on a slippery floor at her workplace. Marsha is also assigned to Mr. Edwards, a 47-year-old, slightly obese man who is in traction for chronic lower back pain. Mr. Edwards is scheduled for physical therapy later in the day.

3. Susan Billman, RN, is caring for Mr. Jackson, a 70-year-old obese man who had thoracic surgery 2 days ago. He continues to have intravenous therapy, but his PCA pump for analgesia was removed 6 hours ago and he has received one dose of Meperidine, 50 mg IM, 1 hour ago. He puts his call light on and says to the nurse, "I am really hurting. Can't you give me something else for the pain?"

4. After her hip replacement, Monica is fearful of using the PCA pump. She asks for q3 hours IM injections of her narcotic analgesic. How can you assess Monica's understanding of the PCA method of pain control? What information does Monica need to have to make this decision?

■ Lippincott Williams & Wilkins Multimedia Resources

McCaffery Pain Library, video (1994)
McCaffery on Pain, video (1992)
McCaffery: Contemporary Issues in Pain Management, video (1994)
Pain Management, CD-ROM (2000)

■ Internet Resources

Pain: www.pain.com
Pain Management: www.aapainmanage.org
Pain Medication: www.painmed.org
Pain Nurses: www.aspm.org

CHAPTER 22

Caring for Clients With Fluid, Electrolyte, and Acid-Base Imbalances

CHAPTER OVERVIEW

Approximately 60% of the adult human body is water, and there is a continuous movement of fluid and exchange of chemicals within the body. Three chemicals—electrolytes, acids, and bases—are involved in the translocation. Osmosis (the movement of water through a semipermeable membrane) helps with fluid distribution. Fluid imbalances include fluid volume deficit, fluid volume excess, and third-spacing. Electrolyte imbalances include hyponatremia, hypernatremia, hypokalemia, hyperkalemia, hypocalcernia, hypercalcemia, hypomagnesemia, and hypermagnesemia. Acid-base imbalances include metabolic acidosis, metabolic alkalosis, respiratory acidosis, and respiratory alkalosis. Nursing management includes early detection of fluid, electrolyte, acid, or base imbalances, assistance with data collection and the collection of appropriate specimens, and implementation and evaluation of medical therapies to correct the imbalances.

KEY TERMS

Acidosis	Filtration
Acids	Generalized edema
Active transport	Hemoconcentration
Alkalosis	Hemodilution
Anion gap	Hypervolemia
Anion gap	Hypovolemia
Anions	Interstitial fluid
Atrial natriuretic peptide	Intracellular fluid
Baroreceptors	Intravascular fluid
Bases	Ions
Bicarbonate-carbonic acid buffer system	Osmoreceptors
	Osmosis
Cations	Passive diffusion
Chvostek's sign	Pitting edema
Circulatory overload	Pitting edema
Compensation	Renin-angiotensin-
Dehydration	aldosterone system
Dependent edema	Serum osmolality
Electrolytes	Skin tenting
Extracellular fluid	Third-spacing
Facilitated diffusion	Thirst
	Trousseau's sign

■ Case Studies

1. Sally Abbott, RN, is caring for several clients who are experiencing disturbances in fluid, electrolyte, acid, or base imbalances. Mr. Fredricks, age 76, is diagnosed with malnutrition and hyponatremia; he is currently hospitalized and is receiving an intravenous solution of sodium chloride. Mrs. Simpson, age 80, has multiple fractures from an auto accident and is diagnosed with hypercalcemia; she is receiving Lasix by mouth twice daily. Ms. Lancet, age 15, is diagnosed with anorexia nervosa, malnutrition, and metabolic acidosis. Mr. Fromm, age 17, is diagnosed with hyperthyroidism and metabolic alkalosis. What is the relationship of water to all of these clients and their medical conditions?

2. Robert Cline, RN, is assigned to care for Mr. Peterson, age 83, who has been recently admitted. Mr. Peterson is diagnosed with kidney failure and is scheduled for renal dialysis. During the nursing assessment, Robert observes the following: the client's blood pressure is 190/104, pulse bounding at 110 beats per minute, respirations at 25 per minute, moist breath sounds, and 4+ pitting edema of the legs and ankles. Mr. Peterson tells the nurse that he has gained 5 pounds during the last week and has had difficulty urinating.

3. June Perry, RN, is assigned to care for Peter Samsung, age 7, following a fire in his home that resulted in second- and third-degree burns to 30% of his body. After admission, Peter developed hypocalcaemia as a result of the burns.

4. The nurse is assigned to care for Erma Sendant, age 74, following cardiac bypass surgery. During

the postoperative period, Erma developed pulmonary edema and is now hospitalized on the cardiac unit. Vital signs include B/P = 156/98, breath sounds moist, breathing labored at 16 breaths per minute, and pulse rate at 120 per minute. Erma tells the nurse, "I am too weak to feed myself and I have a headache." She is being treated for respiratory acidosis.

■ Lippincott Williams & Wilkins Multimedia Resources

Arterial Blood Gas Interpretation, CD-ROM (1998)
RxDx: Arterial Blood Gases, CD-ROM (1997)

■ Internet Resources

Critical points: http://udel.edu/~ccannon/activities.html

CHAPTER 23

Caring for Clients in Shock

CHAPTER OVERVIEW

Shock is a life-threatening condition that occurs when arterial blood flow and oxygen delivery to the cells and tissues are not adequate. The four main types of shock are hypovolemic, distributive, obstructive, and cardiogenic. Nursing management of clients in shock includes data gathering; quickly identifying and reporting signs or symptoms of shock; implementing medical therapy, such as intravenous therapy; planning and providing nursing care; and evaluating the client's response to therapies.

KEY TERMS

Adrenocorticotropic hormone	Hypercarbia
Anaerobic metabolism	Hypovolemic shock
Anaphylactic shock	Hypoxia
Antidiuretic hormone	Irreversible stage
Cardiac output	Ischemia
Cardiogenic shock	Neurogenic shock
Catecholamines	Obstructive shock
Colloid solutions	Oliguria
Compensation stage	Positive inotropic agents
Corticosteroid hormones	Renin-angiotensin-aldosterone system
Crystalloid solutions	Septic shock
Distributive shock	Shock
Endotoxins	Vasopressors

■ Case Studies

1. The nurse is working in the emergency room when a client is admitted on a stretcher with a diagnosis of hypovolemic shock following a severe automobile accident. On arrival, the client's blood pressure is 70/40, pulse is 110 beats per minute, and respirations are at 16 breaths per minute. The client's skin is pale, cool, and somewhat clammy. Intravenous therapy has been initiated by the paramedics in the ambulance en route to the hospital.

2. The nurse is caring for Mrs. Lance following the delivery of a full-term infant weighing 9 lb, 4 oz. The client had significant blood loss after the delivery because the infant was so large. In the recovery room, the nurse plans to assess the client every 15 minutes for at least 1 hour.

3. The nurse is caring for two clients diagnosed with shock. The first client, Mr. Rowe, age 78, is diagnosed with hypovolemic shock from a gunshot wound. He is to be given intravenous dopamine. The second client, Mrs. Josephs, age 65, is diagnosed with cardiogenic shock and is to be given intravenous digoxin.

■ Lippincott Williams & Wilkins Multimedia Resources

Arterial Blood Gas Interpretation, CD-ROM (1998)
RxDx: Arterial Blood Gases, CD-ROM (1997)

■ Internet Resources

Emergency Room Nursing Association:
www.ena.org

CHAPTER 24

Caring for Clients Requiring Intravenous Therapy

CHAPTER OVERVIEW

Intravenous therapy is the parenteral administration of fluids and additives into a vein. It is used to maintain or restore fluid balance when oral replacement is not sufficient or possible. Additives such as electrolytes, vitamins, antibiotics, or other drugs may be given by this route. Blood and blood products are also administered this way. Nurses must be specially skilled to perform venipuncture and administer products by this route. Assessment for untoward results is essential because infection, infiltration, thrombosis, and fluid overload can occur.

KEY TERMS

Blood products
Central venous infusions
Colloid solutions
Drop factors
Drop size
Electronic infusion device
Emulsion
Hypertonic solution
Hypotonic solution
Infusion pump
In-line filter
Intravenous (IV) therapy
Isotonic solution
Macrodrip tubing
Medication lock
Microdrip tubing

Midclavicular catheter
Packed cells
Peripheral venous sites
Phlebitis
Plasma expanders
Pressure infusion sleeve
Primary tubing
Secondary tubing
Total parenteral nutrition
Unvented tubing
Venipuncture
Vented tubing
Volumetric controller
Whole blood
Y-administration tubing

■ Case Studies

1. The nurse is caring for Mrs. Dillman, age 76, who is recovering from chest surgery. The client is to have an IV of lactated Ringer's solution started. The doctor's order reads, "Lactated Ringer's solution IV, 1000 mL over 8 hours." The tubing has a drop factor of 15 gtt/mL.

2. The nurse is caring for Mr. Jones, age 17, following arthroscopic surgery on his left knee. The client is receiving 5% dextrose IV in his right cephalic vein. The nurse plans to assess this client, paying special attention to the IV therapy and the IV site.

2. The nurse is caring for two clients who are receiving IV therapy. Mrs. Patterson, age 70, has just received one unit of packed cells (blood) because her hernatocrit decreased after her surgery. The other client, Mr. Ransom, age 50, is receiving D5W IV following ankle surgery. The nurse plans to assess both clients for complications related to the IV therapy.

■ Lippincott Williams & Wilkins Multimedia Resources

IV Equipment, video (2000)
Administering Peripheral IV Therapy, video (2000)
Administering Central IV Therapy, video (2000)

■ Internet Web Resources

Intravenous Therapies:
www.cc.nih.gov/nurisng/medfsyip.html

CHAPTER 25

Caring for Perioperative Clients

CHAPTER OVERVIEW

The term "perioperative" is used to describe the entire span of a surgical experience and includes the preoperative phase, the operative phase, and the postoperative phase. Surgeries may be diagnostic, exploratory, curative, palliative, or cosmetic. Surgeries may also be classified as emergency, urgent, required, or elective. All surgeries carry potential risk factors and complications. Nurses play an important role with preoperative, operative, and postoperative clients both in the acute care setting and in the outpatient setting.

KEY TERMS

Anesthesia	Malignant hyperthermia
Anesthesiologist	Paralytic ileus
Anesthetist	Perioperative
Conscious sedation	Phlebothrombosis
Dehiscence	Postoperative
Embolus	Preoperative
Evisceration	Surgical asepsis
Intraoperative	Thrombophlebitis

■ Case Studies

1. Judy Pease, RN, is working the evening shift on a surgical unit of the hospital. She is caring for Mr. Billman, age 64, who is admitted for cardiac surgery. She notes that the surgical consent is signed. When the nurse performs the assessment of this client, he says, "I'm not really sure I should even have this surgery. I don't know what they're going to do, and I'm not sure what is expected to happen when I'm done. I'm even wondering how this surgery will affect me in the long term."

2. Sara Evans, RN, is caring for Mrs. Maxwell, age 59, on the evening shift at the local hospital. Mrs. Maxwell is scheduled for bilateral bunionectomies in the morning. While assessing this client, Mrs. Maxwell tells the nurse, "I am really scared about having this surgery. I dread general anesthesia. I lost my nephew and a sister who died unexpectedly during routine surgeries. I really don't know if I should go through with this."

3. The nurse is caring for Mr. Parks, age 65, 5 days after his abdominal surgery. During morning rounds, the nurse begins her assessment of Mr. Parks. He tells the nurse, "I am really nauseated this morning. I was fine yesterday, but today I feel awful. My incision hurts, and I feel as if I am burning up. Can you get me something to help with the nausea?"

■ Lippincott Williams & Wilkins Multimedia Resources

Perioperative Skills, CD-ROM (1999)
Lippincott's Clinical Skills Series: Surgical Care Set, video (1996)
Wound Care, video (1995)

■ Internet Resources

Association of Perioperative Registered Nurses (AORN): www.aorn.org

CHAPTER 26

Caring for Dying Clients

CHAPTER OVERVIEW

Factors with which the nurse needs to be involved when caring for clients who are dying include informing the client, sustaining hope, assisting the client with emotional reactions, and recognizing the client's right to make final decisions. Hospice care provides a home-like environment for clients who are terminally ill. Death gradually occurs over a period of days for the dying client. Pain control is necessary for the dying client, and nurses are responsible to make certain that the client is comfortable. Nurses are also responsible for helping the client and family with spiritual distress; anticipating grief, fear, and hopelessness; and meeting physical needs.

KEY TERMS

Acceptance
Anger
Anticipatory grieving
Bargaining
Denial
Depression
Hospice

Near-death experience
Nearing death awareness
Palliative treatment
Respite care
Waiting for permission
   phenomenon

■ Case Studies

1. A nurse is caring for two clients on the hospice unit. One client is a 26-year-old man who is dying from HIV/AIDS, which he developed after having sexual intercourse with an infected person. The other client is an 84-year-old woman who is dying from pancreatic cancer.

2. Mrs. Altman, age 50, is diagnosed with early breast cancer following a mammogram and a biopsy. The client tells the nurse that she plans to go to Mexico, where she can get coffee enemas and injections with sheep urine for a cure.

3. The nurse is caring for an 88-year-old man who is hospitalized and diagnosed with leukemia. The client tells the nurse, "I want to go home. I want to die at home with my family nearby." The client's wife, age 85, is sitting at his bedside.

■ Multimedia Resources

Gone Tomorrow-AIDS Awareness and AIDS-A Biological Perspective, video. Princeton, NJ: Films for the Humanities and Sciences.
Death and Letting Go-A Hospice Journey, video. Princeton, NJ: Films for the Humanities and Sciences.

■ Internet Resources

Death Education and Counseling: www.adec.org
Grief Links: www.compassionatefriends.org/grieflinks.shtml
Grief Recovery: www.groww.com
Grief Resources: www.aarp.org/griefandloss/
Hospice: www.hospicenet.org

CHAPTER 27

Introduction to the Respiratory System

CHAPTER OVERVIEW

The respiratory system provides oxygen for cellular metabolism and removes carbon dioxide, the waste product. The system is divided into upper and lower airways. Ventilation is the act of moving air in and out of the respiratory tract. Alveolar respiration is the exchange of oxygen for carbon dioxide at the cellular level. Nurses may assist with and/or explain many diagnostic tests to clients and observe for untoward effects.

KEY TERMS

Adenoids	Mediastinum
Alveolus (pl. alveoli)	Nasal septum
Bronchioles	Oropharynx
Bronchus (pl. bronchi)	Paranasal sinuses
Carina	Parietal pleura
Parietal pleura	Perfusion
Cilia	Pharynx
Diaphragm	Pleura
Diffusion	Pleural space
Epiglottis	Respiration
Ethmoidal sinuses	Sphenoidal sinuses
Frontal sinuses	Tonsils
Glottis	Trachea
Hilus	Turbinates (chonchae)
Interstitium	Ventilation
Larynx	Visceral pleura
Lungs	Vocal cords
Maxillary sinuses	

■ Case Study

The nurse is caring for a male client, age 46, who had a laryngoscopy and mediastinoscopy 1 hour ago. The nurse plans to assess the client for possible complications following the procedures.

■ Lippincott Williams & Wilkins Multimedia Resources

Arterial Blood Gas Interpretation, CD-ROM (1998)
Auscultation Skills: Breath and Heart Sounds, CD-ROM (2001)
Auscultation of Breath Sounds, CD-ROM (1998)
Performing Head-to-Toe Assessment, video (2000)
Performing Respiratory Assessment, video (2000)
RxDx: Arterial Blood Gases, CD-ROM (1997)

■ Internet Resources

American Lung Association: www.lungusa.org

CHAPTER 28

Caring for Clients With Upper Respiratory Disorders

CHAPTER OVERVIEW

The most common upper airway disorders are infectious and inflammatory. Upper respiratory disorders include rhinitis, pharyngitis, tonsillitis, adenoiditis, peritonsillar abscess, laryngitis, structural disorders, trauma and obstructional disorders, and malignancies. Nurses who care for clients who have upper respiratory disorders, who need surgical treatment for respiratory conditions, or who have laryngectornies or tracheostomies must provide client and family teaching, prevent infections, and provide emotional support and reassurance.

KEY TERMS

Adenoidectomy	Nasal polyps
Adenoiditis	Peritonsillar abscess
Aphonia	Phyarngitis
Coryza	Rhinorrhea
Deviated septum	Sinusitis
Epistaxis	Stridor
Hemoptysis	Tonsillectomy
Hypertrophied turbinates	Tonsillitis
Laryngitis	Tracheostomy
Laryngoscopy	Tracheotomy

■ Case Studies

1. The nurse in a clinic is caring for a client diagnosed with severe pharyngitis, and the culture reveals group A beta-hemolytic *Streptococcus*. The client is given a prescription for oral penicillin, 500 mg, four times a day.

2. The nurse in the critical care unit is caring for Mr. Adams, who has an endotracheal tube in place. The client is alert and appears to want to communicate. He has an intravenous line in his right hand and is in a low Fowler's position.

3. The nurse is at home when a neighbor calls. The neighbor tells the nurse that she has had a nosebleed for the last half hour and asks the nurse to come to her house.

4. The nurse is caring for Mr. Jilton, age 60, who is scheduled for a partial laryngectomy. The nurse is planning to provide preoperative instructions and postoperative teaching.

■ Lippincott Williams & Wilkins Multimedia Resources

Arterial Blood Gas Interpretation, CD-ROM (1998)
Auscultation Skills: Breath and Heart Sounds, CD-ROM (2001)
Auscultation of Breath Sounds, CD-ROM (1998)
Performing Head-to-Toe Assessment, video (2000)
Performing Respiratory Assessment, video (2000)
RxDx: Arterial Blood Gases, CD-ROM (1997)

■ Internet Resources

Allergic and Nonallergic Rhinitis: www.njc.org
Larynxlink: www.larynxlink.com
NIH Clinical Center Nursing Department SOP: Care of the Patient With a Tracheostomy: www.cc.nih.gov/nursing/trach.html

CHAPTER 29

Caring for Clients With Lower Respiratory Disorders

CHAPTER OVERVIEW

Disorders of the lower respiratory tract include bronchitis, pneumonia, pleurisy, pleural effusion, empyema, influenza, tuberculosis, obstructive pulmonary disease, bronchiectasis, atelectasis, emphysema, asthma, sleep apnea syndrome, occupational lung diseases, and respiratory failure. Nurses caring for clients with these conditions may be involved in providing health teaching, preoperative teaching, and postoperative care. These clients require careful monitoring as acute respiratory failure may develop. Nurses who are caring for clients with malignant tumors are involved with the client and family related to death and dying issues, physical, and spiritual care.

KEY TERMS

Acute bronchitis
Asbestosis
Asthma
Atelectasis
Bronchiectasis
Chronic bronchitis
Chronic obstructive
   pulmonary disease
Cystic fibrosis
Emphysema
Empyema
Flail chest
Hemoptysis
Hemothorax
Influenza
Lobectomy
Lung abscess
Orthopnea
Pleural effusion
Pleurisy
Pneumonectomy
Pneumonia
Pneumoconiosis
Pneumothorax
Polysomnography
Pulmonary contusion
Pulmonary edema
Pulmonary embolism
Pulmonary hypertension
Segmental resection
Septicemia
Silicosis
Sleep apnea syndrome
Subcutaneous emphysema
Thoracotomy
Tracheitis
Tracheobronchitis
Tuberculosis
Wedge resection

■ Case Studies

1. The nurse is caring for a male client on the second postoperative day following cholecystectomy. When the nurse enters the room, the client tells the nurse that he is having trouble breathing and has pain. The nurse plans to assess the client before contacting the physician.

2. The nurse is caring for a client with a history of asthma who has been admitted to the hospital because of uncontrolled diabetes mellitus. The nurse plans to perform the initial admission nursing history and physical assessment.

■ Lippincott Williams & Wilkins Multimedia Resources

Arterial Blood Gas Interpretation, CD-ROM (1998)
Auscultation Skills: Breath and Heart Sounds, CD-ROM (2001)
Auscultation of Breath Sounds, CD-ROM (1998)
Performing Head-To-Toe Assessment, Video (2000)
Performing Respiratory Assessment, Video (2000)
RxDx: Arterial Blood Gases, CD-ROM (1997)

■ Internet Resources

Asthma: www.allergy.mcg.edu/roleAll/outcome.html
Pneumonia and the Elderly:
   www.RespiratoryCare.medscape.com/Home/Topis/
   RespiratoryCare/RespiratoryCare.html
Tuberculosis: www.thoracic.org

CHAPTER 30

Introduction to the Cardiovascular System

CHAPTER OVERVIEW

The cardiovascular system is composed of the heart, major blood vessels, and a vast network of smaller peripheral blood vessels. The myocardium is the muscular layer of the heart. Heart contraction is called systole, and relaxation of the heart is called diastole. Nursing assessments that are essential when caring for cardiac clients include vital signs, presence of pain, peripheral pulses, heart sounds, and presence of edema. While caring for a client who is undergoing diagnostic testing, the nurse is responsible for performing a comprehensive health assessment, health teaching, monitoring the client during the testing, and reporting any unusual findings or symptoms of cardiac decompensation.

KEY TERMS

Angiocardiography	Excitability
Aortography	Hemodynamic monitoring
Arrhythmias	Isoenzyme
Arteriography	Left ventricular
Automaticity	end-diastolic pressure
Baroreceptors	Nomogram
Cardiac index	Phonocardiography
Cardiac output	Polarization
Central venous pressure	Pulmonary capillary
Chemoreceptors	wedge pressure
Conductivity	Refractory period
Contractility	Repolarization
Depolarization	Rhythmicity
Dysrhythmias	Starling's law
Echocardiography	Stroke volume
Electron beam computed	Telemetry
tomography	Transesophageal
Electrocardiography	echocardiography
Electrophysiology	

■ Case Studies

1. A nurse is caring for Mr. Thurman, who is scheduled to have a pulmonary artery catheter inserted. The client's wife asks the nurse, "What is this catheter for, and what will it do once it is in place?"

2. The nurse is caring for a client who is undergoing cardiac stress testing. During the test, the client complains of pain and becomes cyanotic and short of breath.

■ Lippincott Williams & Wilkins Multimedia Resources

12-Lead ECG Interpretation, CD-ROM (1998)
AACN Clinical Simulations: Cardiovascular System II, CD-ROM (1998)
Auscultation Skills: Breath and Heart Sounds, CD-ROM (2001)
Cardiovascular Nursing Videos, video (1992)
Essentials of Cardiac Rhythm Recognition, CD-ROM (1996)
Interactive Electrocardiography, CD-ROM (2000)
Mastering 12-Lead ECGs, video (2000)
Mediclip Clinical Cardiopulmonary Images, CD-ROM (1997)
Nursing Care of Central Venous Catheters, video (1996)
Performing Cardiac Assessment, video (2000)
Reading ECG Rhythm Strips, video (2000)

■ Internet Resources

American Heart Association: www.americanheart.org
Critical Care: www.aacn.org

CHAPTER 31

Caring for Clients With Infectious and Inflammatory Disorders of the Heart and Blood Vessels

CHAPTER OVERVIEW

Inflammatory conditions of the heart include rheumatic fever, infective endocarditis, myocarditis, and pericarditis. Inflammatory disorders of the peripheral blood vessels include thrombophlebitis, and thromboangiitis obliterans (Buerger's disease). Nursing care of clients experiencing these disorders include frequent specific assessments, such as checking Homans' sign; examining the skin, nails, and extremities; administering antioagulants and analgesics; preventing tissue injury; facilitating circulation; and health teaching.

KEY TERMS

Cardiac tamponade
Cardiomyopathy
Carditis
Decortication
Deep vein thrombosis
Doppler ultrasound
Effusion
Emboli
Homans' sign
Hypertrophic cardio-
  myopathy
Impedance plethys-
  mography
Infective endocarditis
Intermittent claudication
Murmur
Myocardial disarray
Myocarditis
Pericardiectomy
Pericardiocentesis
Pericardiostomy

Pericarditis
Petechiae
Plication procedure
Polyarthritis
Postphlebitic syndrome
Precordial pain
Pulmonary embolus
Pulsus paradoxus
Rheumatic carditis
Splinter hemorrhages
Sympathectomy
Syncope
Thrombectomy
Thromboangiitis obliterans
Thrombophlebitis
Vena caval filter
Vena caval plication
  procedure
Venography
Ventriculomyomectomy
Virchow's triad

■ Case Studies

1. A male client visits the clinic and tells the nurse that he has intermittent, cramplike pain after walking; pain when his legs are elevated; and cold, numb feet. The nurse observes several dry ulcerations on the client's feet.

2. A nurse is caring for a female client on prolonged antibiotic therapy for endocarditis with valve involvement. The client tells the nurse, "I am so bored. Why do I need to be on these antibiotics for so long? I don't understand why I just can't go home."

■ Lippincott Williams & Wilkins Multimedia Resources

AACN Clinical Simulations: Cardiovascular System II, CD-ROM (1998)
Auscultation Skills: Breath and Heart Sounds, CD-ROM (2001)
Cardiovascular Nursing Videos, video (1992)
Mediclip Clinical Cardiopulmonary Images, CD-ROM (1997)
Performing Cardiac Assessment, video (2000)
Performing Head-to-Toe Assessment, video (2000)

■ Internet Resources

Buerger's Disease: http://vasculitis.med.jhu.edu/buerger.htm
Cardiomyopathy: www.bu.edu/cohis/cardvasc/heart/cardmyop.htm

CHAPTER 32

Caring for Clients With Valvular Disorders of the Heart

CHAPTER OVERVIEW

Common cardiac valve disorders include aortic stenosis, aortic insufficiency, mitral stenosis, mitral insufficiency, and mitral valve prolapse. These disorders can be diagnosed by echocardiography, chest radiography, and cardiac catheterization. Symptoms include abnormal heart sounds, point of maximal impulse (PMI) displacement, changes in peripheral pulse quality, tachyarrhythmias, syncope, and chest pain. Nursing care of these clients includes comprehensive cardiopulmonary assessment, promotion of adequate circulation and oxygenation, administration of medications, supportive measures to alleviate anxiety, and health teaching.

KEY TERMS

Annuloplasty	Mitral valve prolapse
Aortic regurgitation	syndrome
Aortic stenosis	Point of maximal impulse
Balloon valvuloplasty	Pulmonary hypertension
Commissures	Sequela
Mitral regurgitation	Valvular incompetence
Mitral stenosis	Valvular regurgitation
Mitral valve prolapse	Water-hammer pulse

■ Case Studies

1. A nurse is employed on the cardiac unit of the local hospital and is assigned to care for the following clients: Mrs. Juno, age 27, diagnosed with aortic valve stenosis; Mr. Carter, age 55, diagnosed with mitral valve stenosis; Ms. Louter, age 66, diagnosed with aortic valve insufficiency; and Mr. Milton, age 77, diagnosed with mitral valve insufficiency.

2. The nurse is preparing to admit Mrs. Abrams, age 60, who is being admitted to a semiprivate room with a diagnosis of mitral valve stenosis. The client in the next bed, Mrs. Prescott, age 78, has a diagnosis of tracheobronchitis and has a humidifier next to her bed in addition to numerous aerosol treatments.

■ Lippincott Williams & Wilkins Multimedia Resources

AACN Clinical Simulations: Cardiovascular System II, CD-ROM (1998)
Auscultation Skills: Breath and Heart Sounds, CD-ROM (2001)
Cardiovascular Nursing Videos, video (1992)
Mastering 12-Lead EKG, video (2000)
Performing Cardiac Assessment, video (2000)
Performing Head-to-Toe Assessment, video (2000)
Reading ECG Rhythm Strips, video (2000)

■ Internet Resources

American Heart Association:
   www.americanheart.org
Cardiac Valve Disorders:
   www.swflheartsurgery.com/valve.htm

Caring for Clients With Disorders of Coronary and Peripheral Blood Vessels

CHAPTER OVERVIEW

Cardiovascular disease is the leading cause of death for both men and women in the United States. Disorders of coronary and peripheral blood vessels include arteriosclerosis, atherosclerosis, coronary artery disease, myocardial infarction, Raynaud's disease, thrombosis, phlebothrombosis, embolism, varicose veins, and aneurysms. Nursing management of clients experiencing these conditions includes performing comprehensive cardiovascular assessments, managing the client's pain, teaching the client (preoperatively and postoperatively), administering medications, monitoring laboratory studies, increasing cardiopulmonary circulation, controlling blood pressure, and counseling the client on proper nutrition.

KEY TERMS

Aneurysm
Angina pectoris
Apolipoproteins
Arteriosclerosis
Atherectomy
Atheroma
Atherosclerosis
Bruit
Cardiac rehabilitation
Cholesterol
Coronary artery bypass
   graft
Coronary artery disease
Coronary occlusion
Coronary stent
Coronary thrombosis
Embolus
Enhanced external
   counterpulsation
High-density lipoproteins
Homocysteine
Hyperlipidemia
Infarct

Ischemia
Laser angioplasty
Low-density lipoproteins
Neoangiogenesis
Percutaneous transluminal
   coronary angioplasty
Peripheral vascular disease
Phlebothrombosis
Plaque
Phytoestrogens
Subendocardial infarction
Thrombolytic agents
Thrombosis
Thrombus
Transmyocardial
   revascularization
Topical hyperbaric oxygen
Varicose veins
Vein ligation
Vein stripping
Venous insufficiency
Venous reflux
Venous stasis ulcer

■ Case Studies

1. A 47-year-old man presents in the emergency room complaining of substernal chest pain. The client is diaphoretic and has a history of angina. The nurse plans to perform a nursing history and comprehensive physical assessment of the client.

2. Mrs. Jewel, age 32, visits the client for a routine visit. She had been diagnosed with Raynaud's disease several years ago. Mrs. Jewel tells the clinic nurse, "This winter has been unbelievable...all of this snow and icy weather really get to me. My hands and feet have just felt awful during this bad weather. It seems that the attacks are coming more frequently than ever."

3. The nurse is caring for Mrs. Washington, age 44, following surgery for varicose veins. The nurse is planning for the initial postoperative assessment of the client following a short stay in the hospital's recovery room.

■ Lippincott Williams & Wilkins Multimedia Resources

AACN Clinical Simulations: Cardiovascular System II, CD-ROM (1998)
Auscultation Skills: Breath and Heart Sounds, CD-ROM (2001)
Cardiovascular Nursing Videos, video (1992)
Mediclip Clinical Cardiopulmonary Images, CD-ROM (1997)
Performing Cardiac Assessment, video (2000)
Performing Head-to-Toe Assessment, video (2000)

■ Internet Resources

Cardiovascular Disease:
   www.bu.edu/cohis/cardvasc/cvd
Raynaud's Disease: www.nlm.nih.gov/medlineplus/
   raynaudsdisease.html
Varicose Veins:
   www.bu.edu/cohis/cardvasc/vessel/vein/
   varicose.htm

CHAPTER 34

Caring for Clients With Cardiac Dysrhythmias

CHAPTER OVERVIEW

Common cardiac arrhythmias include sinus bradycardia, atrial fibrillation and atrial flutter, heart block, premature ventricular contractions, ventricular tachycardia and fibrillation, and cardiac arrest. Arrhythmias may be treated with medications, a pacemaker, cardioversion, and defibrillation. Nursing management of clients with arrhythmias includes monitoring and documenting symptoms, monitoring treatment and compliance by the client, and documenting responses to therapies.

KEY TERMS

Asystole
Atrial fibrillation
Atrial flutter
Automatic implanted
   cardiac defibrillator
Bigeminy
Bradydysrhythmia
Chemical cardioversion
Couplets
Defibrillation
Demand (or synchronous)
   mode pacemaker
Dysrhythmia
Ectopic site
Elective electrical
   cardioversion
Fixed-rate (or asynchronous)
   mode pacemaker

Heart block
Implanted pacemaker
Maze procedure
Multifocal PVC
Pacemaker
Premature atrial contraction
Premature ventricular
   contraction
Radiofrequency catheter
   ablation
R on T phenomenon
Sinus bradycardia
Sinus tachycardia
Tachydysrhythmia
Transcutaneous pacemaker
Transvenous pacemaker
Ventricular fibrillation
Ventricular tachycardia

■ Case Studies

1. A client who was diagnosed with atrial fibrillation 2 weeks ago and prescribed ibutilide (Corvert) visits the clinic for a routine visit. The client tells the nurse that he has been taking the medication faithfully as prescribed for the last 2 weeks.

2. The nurse is working on a cardiac rehabilitation unit when a "code blue" is called. The client is experiencing a cardiac arrest, and the resuscitation team has arrived. The nurse is responsible for documenting the cardiopulmonary resuscitative efforts.

■ Lippincott Williams & Wilkins Multimedia Resources

AACN Clinical Simulations: Cardiovascular System II, CD-ROM (1998)
Cardiovascular Nursing Videos, video (1992)
Mastering 12-Lead EKG, video (2000)
Performing Cardiac Assessment, video (2000)
Reading ECG Rhythm Strips, video (2000)

■ Internet Resources

American Heart Association:
   www.americanheart.org
Cardiac Dysrhythmias: www.cardionetics.com

CHAPTER 35

Caring for Clients With Hypertension

CHAPTER OVERVIEW

The term hypertension refers to a sustained elevation of a diastolic arterial pressure of 90 mm Hg or greater, an elevation of systolic arterial pressure of 140 mm Hg or greater, or both. When both vascular damage and heart disease are present along with hypertension, the appropriate term is hypertensive cardiovascular disease. The exact cause of essential hypertension is unknown, but genetic factors may play a role. The cause of secondary hypertension may be due to any primary condition that affects fluid volume, sodium retention, renal function, or any disease process (or medication) that causes vasoconstriction. Nursing care of clients with hypertension includes close blood pressure monitoring; health, nutrition, and medication teaching; and stress reduction and lifestyle improvement teaching.

KEY TERMS

Accelerated hypertension
Diastolic blood pressure
Essential hypertension
Hypernatremia
Hypertension
Hypertensive cardiovascular disease
Hypertensive heart disease

Hypertensive vascular disease
Malignant hypertension
Natriuretic factor
Papilledema
Secondary hypertension
Systolic blood pressure
White-coat hypertension

■ Case Studies

1. A nurse is employed on a cardiovascular unit of an acute care hospital. While caring for Mr. Zenith, age 77, who has been diagnosed with hypertensive cardiovascular disease, the nurse assesses the client's blood pressure. Findings indicate that the blood pressure is 210/112.

2. The nurse is preparing to discharge Mrs. Waters, age 55, from the acute care hospital where the client was treated for essential hypertension. The nurse plans to instruct the client about local support groups and home care follow-up.

■ Lippincott Williams & Wilkins Multimedia Resources

AACN Clinical Simulations: Cardiovascular System II, CD-ROM (1998)
Cardiovascular Nursing Videos, video (1992)
Performing Cardiac Assessment, video (2000)

■ Internet Resources

American Heart Association: www.americanheart.org
American Society of Hypertension: www.ash-us.org
Patient resources: www.pslgroup.com/ hypertension.htm
World Hypertension League: www.mco.edu/org/whl

CHAPTER 36

Caring for Clients With Heart Failure

■ Chapter Overview

Heart failure is a condition that exists when the heart is unable to pump a sufficient amount of blood to meet the body's metabolic needs. Left- or right-sided heart failure or pulmonary edema may be present. In response to low cardiac output, the body begins compensatory mechanisms, which include transitory increased blood pressure, decreased blood flow to the kidneys, hypotension, increased stimulation of rennin-angiotensin-aldosterone secretion, and shunting of the blood to the heart and brain. Nursing care of these clients includes oxygenation, administration of medications, preoperative and postoperative care, monitoring of vital signs and serum electrolytes, monitoring of intake and output, and health teaching.

KEY TERMS

Acute heart failure	Hemoptysis
Afterload	Intra-aortic balloon pump
Aldosterone	Left-sided heart failure
Angiogenesis	Myocardial oxygen demand
Cardiogenic shock	Orthopnea
Cardiac resynchronization therapy	Paroxysmal nocturnal dyspnea
Cardiomyoplasty	Pitting edema
Chronic heart failure	Preload
Congestive heart failure	Pulmonary edema
Cor pulmonale	Pulmonary hypertension
Digitalization	Pulmonary vascular bed
Exertional dyspnea	Renin
Heart failure	Right-sided heart failure
Hemopump	Ventricular assist device

■ Case Studies

1. A nurse is employed on the cardiovascular unit of the hospital. The nurse is assigned to care for Mr. Adams, age 66, diagnosed with left-sided heart failure, and Ms. Jenkins, age 74, diagnosed with right-sided heart failure.

2. The nurse is planning to assess the following clients: Mr. Broman, age 75, diagnosed with right-sided heart failure; and Mrs. Contrel, age 84, diagnosed with left-sided heart failure.

3. The nurse is caring for Mrs. Shortling, age 88, diagnosed with heart failure. The nurse assesses the client and determines the following: B/P = 110/50, pulse = 100, temperature = 99, respirations = 42/min, crackles in both bases of lungs, complaint of nausea, pulse oximeter reading of 89%, enlarged, soft abdomen.

■ Lippincott Williams & Wilkins Multimedia Resources

AACN Clinical Simulations: Cardiovascular System II, CD-ROM (1998)
Auscultation Skills: Breath and Heart Sounds, CD-ROM (2001)
Cardiovascular Nursing Videos, video (1992)
Mediclip Clinical Cardiopulmonary Images, CD-ROM (1997)
Nursing Care of Central Venous Catheters, video (1996)
Performing Cardiac Assessment, video (2000)
Performing Head-To-Toe Assessment, video (2000)

■ Internet Resources

Information: www.heartinfo.org
Heart Disease: www.medstudents.com.br/cardio/cardio3.htm
Congestive Heart Failure: www.nhibi.nih.gov/index.htm
Heart Failure: www.medgraph.com/aboutheart.html

CHAPTER 37

Caring for Clients Undergoing Cardiovascular Surgery

CHAPTER OVERVIEW

The techniques for mechanically circulating and oxygenating blood outside of the body, or extracorporeal circulation (cardiopulmonary bypass), were developed in the 1960s. Cardiovascular surgeries include repair of valves by commissurotomy, coronary artery bypass graft, repair of aneurysms, removal of tumors, repair of trauma, heart transplantation, and repair of central or peripheral vascular surgical procedures, such as embolectomies. Nursing care of clients undergoing heart surgery includes preoperative preparation and teaching; intraoperative monitoring; postoperative care, which includes careful monitoring of cardiovascular status; neurologic assessments; and client and family teaching.

KEY TERMS

Annuloplasty
Cardioplegia
Cardiopulmonary bypass
Commissurotomy
Coronary artery bypass graft
Embolectomy
Endarterectomy
Extracorporeal circulation
Myocardial revascularization
Thrombectomy
Valvuloplasty

■ Case Studies

1. A nurse is caring for Mr. Dowdy, age 66, following coronary artery bypass graft surgery. The nursing assessment finds the following: leg pain, which the client reports as 8 on a scale of 1 to 10; respirations of 30 breaths per minute at rest; dried blood on the thoracic dressing; sore throat after being weaned from mechanical ventilation; and concern that he has not had a bowel movement in 3 days.

2. A nurse is caring for Mrs. Twine, age 70, following cardiac surgery and a thoracotomy. Nursing assessment reveals the following: weak cough, shallow respirations, and diminished breath sounds.

■ Lippincott Williams & Wilkins Multimedia Resources

AACN Clinical Simulations: Cardiovascular System II, CD-ROM (1998)
Cardiovascular Nursing Videos, video (1992)
Mediclip Clinical Cardiopulmonary Images, CD-ROM (1997)
Performing Cardiac Assessment, video (2000)
Performing Head-to-Toe Assessment, video (2000)

■ Internet Resources

Journal of Thoracic and Cardiovascular Surgery: www.harcourthealth.com/jtws/

CHAPTER 38

Introduction to the Hematopoietic and Lymphatic Systems

CHAPTER OVERVIEW

The term "hematopoiesis" means the manufacture and development of blood cells. While most blood cells are produced in the bone marrow, the lymphatic system and the thymus gland also play a role. Nursing care of clients with disorders of the hematopoietic and lymphatic systems includes conducting an accurate health history and physical assessment, teaching related to diagnostic tests, monitoring laboratory values, assisting with bone marrow aspirations, and health teaching following diagnosis of the disorder.

KEY TERMS

Agranulocytes	Leukocytosis
Basophils	Leukopenia
Erythrocytes	Lymph
Erythropoiesis	Lymph nodes
Erythropoietin	Lymphatics
Granulocytes	Lymphocytes
Hematopoiesis	Neutrophils
Hemoglobin	Phagocytosis
Leukocytes	Plasma
	Pluripotential stem cells

■ Case Studies

1. A nurse is planning a presentation to a group of high school students on the topic of "Anatomy and Physiology of the Hematopoietic System."
2. A nurse is caring for Mr. Andrews, age 59, who is scheduled for a bone marrow aspiration. The nurse will assist the physician during the procedure.
3. A nurse is caring for Mrs. Michaels, age 71. The client's laboratory studies reveal the following: platelets, 80,000; RBC, 2.4 million; and WBC, 24,500.

■ Lippincott Williams & Wilkins Multimedia Resources

AACN Clinical Simulations: Hematologic System, CD-ROM (1999)
Atlas of Blood Pathology, CD-ROM (1997)
Atlas of Lymph Node Pathology, CD-ROM (1997)
Hematology Atlas, CD-ROM (1996)
Transfusing Blood Safely, video (1992)

■ Internet Resources

Lymph nodes: http://anatomy.uams.edu/HTMLpages/anatomyhtml/lymph_alpha.html
Stem Cell Transplant: www.itxm.org/Archive/trmus-95.htm

CHAPTER 39

Caring for Clients With Disorders of the Hematopoietic System

CHAPTER OVERVIEW

Blood dyscrasias, abnormalities in the number and types of blood cells, and bleeding disorders develop from both treatable and chronic pathologic processes. Blood dyscrasias include various anemias, polycythemias, leukemias, multiple myelomas, agranulocytosis, pancytopenias, and thrombocytopenias. Nursing care for clients with these disorders includes a thorough history and physical assessment, health teaching, administration of prescribed medications, supportive treatments, promotion of activities to reduce pain or fatigue, institution of neutropenic precautions when necessary, and referral to home care or support groups.

KEY TERMS

Acute chest syndrome	Heme
Agranulocytosis	Leukocytosis
Anemia	Leukopenia
Aplasia	Pancytopenia
Blood dyscrasias	Sickle cell anemia
Coagulopathies	Thrombocytopenia
Erythrocytosis	

■ Case Studies

1. The nurse is caring for the following clients: Mr. Marks, age 54, diagnosed with hypovolemic anemia and shock; Mrs. Andrews, age 32, diagnosed with iron deficiency anemia; Ms. Lewis, age 18, diagnosed with sickle cell anemia; Mr. Putnam, age 88, diagnosed with hemolytic anemia; Mrs. Howard, age 45, diagnosed with thalassemia; Mr. Greene, age 56, diagnosed with pernicious anemia; and Ms. Brown, age 22, diagnosed with folic acid deficiency anemia.

2. The nurse is caring for the following clients: Mrs. York, age 40, diagnosed with iron deficiency anemia; Mr. Banter, age 67, diagnosed with chronic lymphocytic anemia; and Ms. Dillman, age 34, diagnosed with thrombocytopenia.

■ Lippincott Williams & Wilkins Multimedia Resources

AACN Clinical Simulations: Hematologic System, CD-ROM (1999)
Atlas of Blood Pathology, CD-ROM (1997)
Hematology Atlas, CD-ROM (1996)
Transfusing Blood Safely, video (1992)

■ Internet Resources

Anemia: www.anemiacenter.com
Leukemia links: www.acor.org/leukemia/

CHAPTER 40

Caring for Clients With Disorders of the Lymphatic System

CHAPTER OVERVIEW

Lymphatics are a system of vessels that carry fluid from the body tissues to the veins. Lymphatic disorders are infectious, inflammatory, occlusive, or malignant conditions. Examples include lymphedema, lymphangitis, lymphadenitis, infectious mononucleosis, Hodgkin's disease, and non-Hodgkin's lymphoma. Nursing care of these clients includes an accurate and thorough health history and physical assessment, administration of prescribed medications, assistance with biopsies and other medical procedures, maintenance of airway patency, nutritional counseling, supportive treatments, health teaching, and home care referrals or support groups.

KEY TERMS

Epstein-Barr virus	Lymphatics
Hodgkin's disease	Lymphedema
Infectious mononucleosis	Lymphoma
Lymph	Non-Hodgkin's lymphoma
Lymphadenitis	Reed-Sternberg cell
Lymphangitis	

■ Case Studies

1. The nurse is caring for two clients: Mr. Jasper, age 67, diagnosed with lymphedema, and Mrs. Williams, age 83, diagnosed with non-Hodgkin's lymphoma.

2. The nurse is caring for Mrs. Morrow, age 73, diagnosed with lymphedema.

3. The nurse is caring for Mr. Buell, age 65, who has just been diagnosed with Hodgkin's disease.

■ Lippincott Williams & Wilkins Multimedia Resources

Atlas of Blood Pathology, CD-ROM (1997)
Atlas of Lymph Node Pathology, CD-ROM (1997)

■ Internet Resource

Leukemia and Lymphoma Society:
   www.leukemia.org
Lymphoma:
   www.lymphomainfo.nte/nhl/description.html

Introduction to the Immune System

CHAPTER OVERVIEW

Chapter 41 is an introduction to the immune system. The immune response is a target-specific system of defense carried out primarily by lymphocytes. Disorders of this system can be life-threatening.

KEY TERMS

Anergy	Macrophages
Antibodies	Memory cells
Antigens	Microphages
Artificially-acquired	Monocytes
active immunity	Naturally acquired
Cell-mediated response	active immunity
Cytotoxic T cells	Neutrophils
Effector T cells	Passive immunity
Helper T cells	Phagocytosis
Humoral response	Plasma cells
Immune response	Regulator T cells
Immunoglobulins	Stem cells
Lymphokines	Suppressor T cells

■ Case Studies

1. Your friend, Marsha, tells you that her sister has been diagnosed with an immune disorder.

2. The nurse is caring for a newly delivered first-time mother. The mother asks the nurse, "Why should I have my baby immunized?"

3. The nurse is caring for the following clients: Ms. Arks, age 10, who has a hepatitis B vaccine ordered; Mr. Benson, age 2, who has a chickenpox vaccine ordered; and Mrs. Landers, age 40, who has a gamma globulin injection ordered.

4. Kevin Banks is admitted to the medical floor with a diagnosis of hepatitis B. His wife has not been immunized against hepatitis B. What type of immunization would be recommended for her now? How long will the coverage last? What teaching is necessary for Kevin and his wife to protect her at this time?

■ Internet Resources

Immunizations: www.immunize.org
Immunization Schedule: www.cdc.gov
Self-Regulation:
    www.cjnetworks.com/~lifesci/immu.htm

Caring for Clients With Immune-Mediated Disorders

CHAPTER OVERVIEW

Chapter 42 discusses allergic and autoimmune disorders and appropriate nursing care for these clients. Additionally, management of chronic fatigue syndrome, a consequence of immune-mediated disorder, is covered.

KEY TERMS

Anergy	Macrophages
Antibodies	Memory cells
Antigens	Microphages
Artificially acquired active immunity	Monocytes
	Naturally acquired active immunity
Cell-mediated response	
Cytotoxic T cells	Neutrophils
Effector	Passive immunity
T cells	Phagocytosis
Helper T cells	Plasma cells
Humoral response	Regulator T cells
Immune response	Stem cells
Immunoglobulins	Suppressor T cells
Lymphokines	

■ Case Study

1. Jonah has complained of a runny nose, watery eyes, and wheezing for 3 weeks. He will come to the clinic for skin testing for allergies. What teaching does he need prior to his visit? What teaching will he need at his visit? What is the priority nursing diagnosis for Jonah?

■ Internet Resources

Autoimmune Disorders:
   www.hml.org/CHIS/topics/immune.html
Chronic Fatigue Syndrome: www.cfids.org
Latex Allergy: www.latexallergylinks.tripod.com

CHAPTER 43

Caring for Clients With AIDS

CHAPTER OVERVIEW

Chapter 43 explains the infectious and often fatal disorder known as acquired immunodeficiency syndrome (AIDS). AIDS may develop after exposure to human immunodeficiency virus (HIV).

KEY TERMS

Acquired immunodeficiency
  syndrome
Acute retroviral syndrome
Autologous blood
Directed donor blood
Enzyme-linked immuno-
  sorbent assay (ELISA)
Human immunodeficiency
  virus
Integrase
Kaposi's sarcoma
p24 antigen test

Pneumocystic pneumonia
Polymerase chain reaction
  (PCR) test
Protease
Protease inhibitor
Retrovirus
Reverse transcriptase
Reverse transcriptase
  (RT) inhibitor
Reverse transcription
Western blot

■ Case Studies

1. Mr. Young, age 24, has recently been hospitalized with an infection as a result of the AIDS virus. He is preparing to be discharged and desires to go to his parents' home for supportive home care. The parents contact the nurse during a pre-discharge interview, and they tell the nurse that they are fearful about becoming infected if they allow Mr. Young to come home.

2. The nurse is planning a presentation to a group of high school students on the topic of "HIV/AIDS Prevention."

3. The nurse has just administered Morphine sulfate intramuscularly to Mr. Parkman, age 34, diagnosed with a possible peptic ulcer. While trying to place the contaminated needle into the sharps container, the nurse sustains a needle stick.

4. Joseph is a 20-year-old college student who comes to the student health center wanting to be tested for HIV. He is concerned because he recently had a sexual encounter while under the influence of alcohol, and he did not use a condom. What teaching is necessary prior to the counseling? What information does Joseph need to know to prevent HIV transmission? When would you recommend Joseph return for retesting?need to know to prevent HIV transmission? When would you recommend Joseph return for retesting?

■ Internet Resources

AIDS Foundation: www.sonoma-aids.org
AIDS Newsletter: www.hain.org/aidsaction.html
AIDS Statistics:
  www.cdc.gov/nchstp/hiv_aids/stats.htm
AIDS Treatment: www.hivatis.org/atisinfo.html

CHAPTER 44

Introduction to the Nervous System

CHAPTER OVERVIEW

The nervous system is divided into two divisions: the central nervous system (CNS) and the peripheral nervous system. The neuron, or nerve cell, is the basic structure of the nervous system. Impulses travel along neurons by synapses, and transmission of an impulse is accomplished by neurotransmitters. The brain and spinal cord comprise the CNS, and the peripheral nervous system includes all nerves outside the CNS. Nursing care of clients with neurologic disorders includes a complete neurologic and physical examination, recording of vital signs, assistance with diagnostic tests, and client and family teaching. When caring for the older adult, the nurse may find that drug toxicity may be evident when there is a change in mental status, memory may be difficult, and pupillary response may be more sluggish.

KEY TERMS

Acetylcholine	Medulla oblongata
Acetylcholinesterase	Meninges
Arachnoid	Midbrain
Axon	Myelin
Brain stem	Neurilemma
Cauda equina	Neuron
Central nervous system	Neurotransmitter
Cerebellum	Norepinephrine
Cerebrum	Parasympathetic nervous
Corpus callosum	system
Decerebrate posturing	Peripheral nervous system
Decorticate posturing	Pia mater
Dendrites	Pons
Dopamine	Pyramidal
Dura mater	Subarachnoid space
Epinephrine	Sympathetic nervous system
Extrapyramidal	Ventricle

■ Case Studies

1. The nurse is caring for Mrs. Ardor, age 65, following hospitalization with several fractures as a result of an automobile accident. The nurse is preparing to perform a neurologic assessment of the client.

2. The nurse is caring for the following clients: Mr. Minion, age 70, who is scheduled to have a lumbar puncture; Mrs. Aloe, age 55, who is scheduled to have a cerebral angiogram to rule out a brain aneurysm; and Ms. Nightly, age 77, who is scheduled to have a brain scan to rule out a tumor.

■ Lippincott Williams & Wilkins Multimedia Resources

Interactive Neuroanatomy, CD-ROM (2001)
Lippincott's Clinical Care Series: Assessment Set, video (1997)
Neurological Assessment, CD-ROM (1996)
Neuroscience Nursing Videos, video (1995)
Performing Head-to-Toe Assessment, video (2000)
Visual Guide to Physical Examination, A, video (1994)
Whole Brain Atlas, CD-ROM (1999)

■ Internet Resources

Autonomic Nervous System:
www.nda.ox.ac.uk/wfsa/html/u05/u05_010.htm
Brain and Spinal Cord Anatomy:
http://faculty.washington.edu/chudler.introb.htm
Images: www.innerbody.com/image/nervov.html
Nervous System: http://gened.emc.maricopa.edu/
bio/bio101/BIOBK/BiobookNERV.html

Caring for Clients With Central and Peripheral Nervous System Disorders

CHAPTER OVERVIEW

Acute neurologic disorders can be potentially life threatening, whereas chronic neurologic disorders can profoundly affect an individual's quality of life. Acute disorders include increased intracranial pressure, meningitis, encephalitis, Guillain-Barré syndrome, and brain abscess. Chronic disorders include multiple sclerosis, myasthenia gravis, amyotrophic lateral sclerosis (ALS or Lou Gehrig's disease), cranial nerve disorders, Bell's palsy, temporomandibular joint syndrome, Parkinson's disease, Huntington's disease, seizure disorders (e.g., epilepsy), and brain tumors. Nursing care of clients with central and peripheral nervous system disorders includes completing a careful nursing history and physical assessment, notifying the physician if symptoms worsen, assisting with diagnostic testing, monitoring vital signs, administering prescribed medications, monitoring the effects of drug therapy, providing preoperative and postoperative care, ensuring safety and seizure precautions, promoting nutritional intake, and teaching the client and family.

KEY TERMS

Aura	Foramen magnum
Automatisms	Kernig's sign
Bradykinesia	Neuralgia
Brudzinski's sign	Nuchal rigidity
Cheyne-Stokes respirations	Nystagmus
Choreiform movements	Opisthotonos
Convulsion	Papilledema
Cushing's triad	Parkinsonism
Demyelinating disease	Photophobia
Diplopia	Preictal phase
Epilepsy	Ptosis
Fasciculations	Seizure

■ Case Studies

1. The nurse is caring for Mr. Louden, age 45, who is scheduled for an appendectomy. The client tells the nurse that he has a history of epilepsy with tonic-clonic seizures and has been taking Dilantin for the last 5 years.

2. The nurse is caring for Mrs. Zont, age 44, who has just been diagnosed with multiple sclerosis.

3. The nurse is preparing to discharge Mr. Plank, age 77, who has been diagnosed as being in the deteriorating stages of Parkinson's disease. The client's wife (age 75) of 54 years is present and is helping the client prepare for his discharge.

■ Lippincott Williams & Wilkins Multimedia Resources

Interactive Neuroanatomy, CD-ROM (2001)
Neurological Assessment, CD-ROM (1996)
Neuroscience Nursing Videos, video (1995)

■ Internet Resources

Amyotrophic Lateral Sclerosis: www.alsa.org
Bell's Palsy: www.ninds.nih.gove/health_and_medical/disorders/bells_doc.htm
Brain Abscess: www.emedicine.com/emerg/topic67.htm
Brain and Nervous System topics: www.nlm.nih.gov/medlineplus/brainandnervoussystem.html
Brain Tumors: www.abta.org
Encephalitis: http://communities.msn.com/EncephalitisGlobal

Guillain-Barré Syndrome: www.guillain-barre.com

Huntington's Disease: www.hdsa.org

Increased Intracranial Pressure:
http://traumaburn.com/ICP.htm

Meningitis: www.meningitis.org

Multiple Sclerosis: www.nmss.org

Myasthenia Gravis: www.myasthenia.org

Nervous System Diseases:
www.mic.ki.se/Diseases/c10.html

Parkinson's Disease: www.parkinson.org

Seizure Disorders:
www.neurologychannel.com/seizures

Temporomandibular Disorder:
www.floss.com/tmd_temporomandibular_disorder
.htm

Trigeminal Neuralgia: www.tna-support.org

CHAPTER 46

Caring for Clients With Cerebrovascular Disorders

CHAPTER OVERVIEW

Although some cerebrovascular disorders such as a cerebrovascular accident (CVA, stroke) are potentially life-threatening, other cerebrovascular disorders cause tremendous discomfort and can affect the quality of an individual's life. Transient headaches are considered benign, but may have varying degrees of discomfort associated with the conditions. There are three categories of headaches: tension, migraine, and cluster headaches. Cerebrovascular disorders include transient ischemic attacks; these may be a warning of a CVA. Cerebral aneurysms can affect cranial nerve function and may require surgical repair. Nursing care of clients with cerebrovascular disorders includes a thorough history and physical assessment; monitoring of symptoms of worsening conditions; administration of medications; pre- and postoperative care; rehabilitation, referrals and home or long-term care provision; client and family health teaching; promotion of adequate nutrition; and prevention of complications, such as pneumonia and pressure ulcers.

KEY TERMS

Aneurysm	Endarterectomy
Bruit	Expressive aphasia
Cephalalgia	Hemianopia
Cerebral infarction	Hemiplegia
Cerebrovascular accident	Receptive aphasia
Collateral circulation	Transient ischemic attack

■ Case Studies

1. The nurse is having lunch with a friend, who tells her, "I've really been bothered by my migraine headaches lately. Do you have any suggestions?"

2. The nurse has just admitted Mr. Albee, age 79, to the hospital following a cerebrovascular accident (stroke). The nurse plans to develop a plan of care after taking the client's history and physical assessment.

3. The nurse is caring for Mrs. Pinto, age 81, who has been hospitalized and diagnosed with a leaking cerebral aneurysm.

■ Lippincott Williams & Wilkins Multimedia Resources

Interactive Neuoranatomy, CD-ROM (2001)
McCaffery Pain Library, video (1994)
McCaffery on Pain, video (1992)
McCaffery: Contemporary Issues in Pain
    Management, video (1994)
Neurological Assessment, CD-ROM (1996)
Neuroscience Nursing Videos, video (1995)
Pain Management, CD-ROM (2000)

■ Internet Resources

Cerebral Aneurysm: www.ninds.nih.gov/
    health_and_medical/disorders/ceraneur_doc.htm
Cerebrovascular Accident: www.stroke.org
Headaches: www.headaches.org

CHAPTER 47

Caring for Clients With Head and Spinal Cord Trauma

CHAPTER OVERVIEW

Head trauma or injuries can result in brain concussions, contusions, epidural or subdural hematomas, or skull fractures. All head injuries should be regarded as an emergency because head trauma can be life threatening. Spinal cord injuries can result in paralysis or death. Most spinal cord injuries are the result of automobile accidents, although they can also be the result of violence, falls, sports, or miscellaneous injuries. Spinal nerve root compressions include intermedullary lesions that involve the spinal cord or extramedullary lesions that involve the tissues surrounding the spinal cord. Various diagnostic tests are used to confirm head and spinal cord injuries. Nursing care for clients with head or spinal cord injuries includes completing a thorough and accurate health history and physical assessment, providing preoperative and postoperative care, administering prescribed medications, monitoring vital signs and intake and output, assisting with breathing, providing pain management, performing neurologic assessments, monitoring for signs of increased intracranial pressure, assisting with mobility, providing stress and coping mechanisms, and teaching the client and family about the disorder and its management.

KEY TERMS

Autonomic dysreflexia	Intracerebral hematoma
Autoregulation	Intramedullary
Battle's sign	Laminectomy
Cerebral hematoma	Open head injury
Chemonucleolysis	Otorrhea
Closed head injury	Paraplegia
Concussion	Paresthesia
Contrecoup injury	Periorbital ecchymosis
Contusion	Poikilothermia
Coup injury	Rhinorrhea
Craniectomy	Spinal fusion
Cranioplasty	Spinal shock
Craniotomy	Subdural hematoma
Diskectomy	Supratentorial
Epidural hematoma	Tentorium
Extramedullary	Tetraplegia
Halo sign	Uncal herniation
Infratentorial	

■ Case Studies

1. Mr. Mensa, age 36, is brought to the emergency room by ambulance following a motor vehicle accident. The client was not wearing a seat belt, and his head struck the steering wheel of his pickup truck.

2. A nurse makes a home visit to Mrs. Lippman, age 44, who is a paraplegic as a result of a motor vehicle accident.

■ Lippincott Williams & Wilkins Multimedia Resources

Neurological Assessment, CD-ROM (1996)
Neuroscience Nursing Videos, video (1995)
Rehabilitation of the Spine Video Series, video (1998)
Safe Back Workout, video (1998)
Spinal Stabilization, video (1998)

■ Internet Resources

Head Injuries: www.headinjury.com
Spinal Cord Injuries: www.spinalcord.org

CHAPTER 48

Caring for Clients With Neurologic Deficits

CHAPTER OVERVIEW

A neurologic deficit occurs when one or more functions of the central or peripheral nervous system are decreased. Neurologic deficits are divided into three phases: acute, recovery, and chronic. The acute phase usually occurs after sudden neurologic trauma, and the client is typically critically ill. The recovery phase begins when the client's condition is stabilized. In some conditions (e.g., multiple sclerosis), clients experience the chronic phase as their initial symptoms. For other clients, the chronic phase is the period in which their condition shows little or no improvement, becomes stationary, or worsens. Nursing care for clients with these disorders includes a obtaining a complete nursing history and physical assessment with special emphasis on neurologic assessments, promoting elimination, preventing contractures or pressure ulcers, counseling regarding sexual dysfunction, assisting the client or family to cope with the disability, maintaining skin care and hygiene, teaching the client and family, and referring for home care services or support groups.

KEY TERMS

Credé maneuver	Neurologic deficit
Cutaneous triggering	Reflex incontinence

■ Case Studies

1. The nurse is caring for Mrs. Ruby, age 45, who is a paraplegic in the recovery stage. The nurse is planning to teach the client about bowel and bladder training.

2. The nurse is caring for Mr. Scranton, age 80, who suffered a CVA 6 months ago. The client is paralyzed on his right side, is aphasic, and is showing signs of mental changes as a result of the CVA. When the nurse enters the room, the client appears agitated and is making motions with his left hand to various areas of his body, primarily his abdomen.

3. The nurse in a rehabilitation center joins members of the health care team in a clinical conference. The client under discussion is Mr. Cox, age 22, who suffered a spinal cord injury at T-11 and is a paraplegic. The client is severely depressed and withdrawn.

4. The nurse is caring for Mrs. Deems, age 59, who was diagnosed with multiple sclerosis several years ago. Within the past year she has required a wheelchair and has had limited use of her arms. The client has been admitted for a skin graft to a sacral pressure ulcer.

■ Lippincott Williams & Wilkins Multimedia Resources

Neurological Assessment, CD-ROM (1996)
Neuroscience Nursing Videos, video (1995)
Post-Isometric Relaxation Techniques, video (1998)

■ Internet Resource

Aphasia: www.aphasia.org

CHAPTER 49

Caring for Clients With Eye Disorders

CHAPTER OVERVIEW

The eyes are divided into the anterior and posterior chambers and are protected by fat and muscles in the face. Eye examinations and assessments may be done by optometrists and ophthalmologists. These examinations include visual screening, retinoscopy, tonometry, visual field examination, slit lamp examination, retinal angiography, and ultrasonography. Visual disorders include refractive errors, blindness, eye trauma, infectious and inflammatory disorders, macular degeneration, glaucoma, cataracts, retinal detachment, and enucleation. Nursing care for clients experiencing visual disorders includes assisting with visual testing, assisting the newly blind individual to cope with the disability, providing preoperative and postoperative care and teaching, explaining prevention strategies, administering prescribed medications, and teaching the client and family.

KEY TERMS

Accommodation	Keratoplasty
Astigmatism	Myopia
Cataract	Near point
Central vision	Nystagmus
Conjunctivitis	Ophthalmoscopy
Corneal transplantation	Photophobia
Corneal trephine	Presbyopia
Diplopia	Ptosis
Ernmetropia	Refraction
Endophthalmitis	Retinal detachment
Enucleation	Tonometry
Glaucoma	Trabeculoplasty
Hordeolum	Uveitis
Hyperopia	Visual acuity
Intraocular lens implant	Visual field examination
Iridectomy	Visually impaired
Keratitis	

■ Case Studies

1. Mr. Peltier, age 35, visits the clinic for a routine checkup. He tells the nurse that he has had "difficulty seeing lately."

2. Mrs. Ransom, age 34, asks the nurse, "What does 20/200 visual acuity mean?"

3. The nurse is planning to perform an examination of the eyes of Mr. Bilmar, age 60.

4. Mr. Bowlen, age 40, is seen in the emergency room after he was hit with a baseball to his left eye.

5. A mother brings her son, Albert, age 9, to the client for a follow-up visit for treatment for an infectious eye disorder.

6. A 24-year-old friend tells the nurse, "My father had glaucoma and needed treatment."

7. The nurse is caring for Mrs. Cowen, age 77, who is scheduled for a cataract extraction.

■ Lippincott Williams & Wilkins Multimedia Resources

Acland's Video Atlas of Human Anatomy: The Head and Neck, Part I, video (1998)

■ Internet Resources

Blindness and Sports Injuries: www.preventblindness. org/safety/sprtsafe.html
Cataracts: www.indian-river.fl.us/health/ eyedisorders/cataracts.html
Eye and Ear Institute: www.nyee.edu
Glaucoma: www.glaucoma.org

CHAPTER 50

Caring for Clients With Ear Disorders

CHAPTER OVERVIEW

The ear is divided into three areas: the outer, the middle, and the inner sections. Basic hearing acuity tests include observation, otoscopic examination, tuning fork tests, and the Romberg test. Diagnostic studies include audiometry, caloric stimulation tests, and electronystagmography. Hearing impairment may range from mild to profound. Disorders of the external ear include impacted cerumen, foreign bodies in the ear, and otitis externa. Disorders of the middle ear include otitis media and otosclerosis. Disorders of the inner ear include Meniere's disease, which often includes tinnitus. Nursing care of clients with hearing disorders includes taking a thorough nursing history and physical examination, assisting with hearing and diagnostic testing, assisting with communication, administering prescribed medications, teaching preventive techniques such as wearing earplugs, administering preoperative and postoperative care, instituting safety measures, and teaching the client and family about the disorder and its management.

KEY TERMS

Acoustic neuroma	Otitis media
Audiometry	Otosclerosis
Caloric stimulation test	Otoscope
Cochlear implant	Ototoxicity
Conductive hearing loss	Presbycusis
Decibels	Rinne test
Electronystagmography	Romberg test
Labyrinthitis	Sensorineural hearing loss
Mastoidectomy	Sign language
Mastoiditis	Speech reading
Meniere's disease	Stapedectomy
Myringoplasty	Tinnitus
Myringotomy	Tuning fork
Nystagmus	Weber test
Otitis externa	

■ Case Studies

1. The nurse is caring for the following clients: Mr. Partridge, age 65, diagnosed with hearing loss due to impacted cerumen; Mrs. Lance, age 50, diagnosed with otosclerosis and hearing loss; and Mr. Cochran, age 55, diagnosed with hearing loss caused by Meniere's disease.

2. The nurse is caring for Mr. Martin, age 55, who is hospitalized for gallbladder surgery. The client is deaf as a result of congenital deafness and communicates via sign language.

■ Lippincott Williams & Wilkins Multimedia Resources

Acland's Video Atlas of Human Anatomy: The Head and Neck, Part I, video (1998)

■ Internet Resources

Acoustic Neuroma: www.anausa.org
Ear Surgery: www.earsurgery.org
Hearing Loss: www.hearingloss.com
Meniere's Disease: www.menieres.org

CHAPTER 51

Introduction to the Gastrointestinal System and Accessory Structures

CHAPTER OVERVIEW

The gastrointestinal (GI) system can be divided into the upper and lower GI tracts. Accessory structures include the gallbladder, peritoneum, liver, and pancreas. During a physical assessment, the nurse should inspect the client's general appearance; assess the client's skin for color, turgor, and moisture; and examine the client's mouth, abdomen, and anus. Diagnostic studies for GI disorders include radiography and nonradiographic imagery. Gastrointestinal tests include percutaneous liver biopsy and GI endoscopy. Various laboratory tests can be used to confirm GI disorders. General nursing care for clients with suspected GI disorders includes obtaining a thorough history and physical examination; checking vital signs, weight, and height; documenting allergies; observing for rectal bleeding; and teaching the client and family about diagnostic testing and laboratory studies.

KEY TERMS

Barium enema
Barium swallow
Cholangiography
Cholecystography
Colonoscopy
Endoscopic retrograde
    cholangiopancreatography
Enteroclysis
Esophagogastroduo-
    endoscopy
Flexible sigmoidoscopy
Gallbladder series

Lower gastrointestinal
    series
Panendoscopy
Percutaneous liver biopsy
Peristalsis
Proctosigmoidoscopy
PY test
Radionuclide imaging
Small bowel enteroscopy
Ultrasonography
Upper gastrointestinal
    series

■ Case Studies

1. A nurse is caring for two clients: Mr. Samuels, age 66, who is scheduled for a lower GI series, and Mrs. Larson, age 71, who is scheduled for a colonoscopy.

2. A nurse is caring for Mr. Paxton, age 70, who has just had a liver biopsy. During the immediate recovery period, Mr. Paxton's blood pressure drops from 120/77 to 90/54.

■ Lippincott Williams & Wilkins Multimedia Resources

Gastrointestinal Pathology Plus, CD-ROM (1999)
Performing Head-to-Toe Assessment, video (2000)

■ Internet Resources

American Gastroenterology Organization:
    www.gastro.org
GI Disorders:
    www.iffgd.org/GIDisorders/GIMain.html

CHAPTER 52

Caring for Clients With Disorders of the Upper Gastrointestinal Tract

■ Chapter Overview

The process of digestion begins in the mouth and continues in the stomach and small intestine. Disorders of the upper intestinal tract include anorexia, nausea and vomiting, cancer of the oral cavity, gastroesophageal reflux disorder (GERD), esophageal diverticula, hiatal hernia, cancer of the esophagus, gastritis, peptic ulcers, and cancer of the stomach. Medical and surgical management of these disorders include intravenous therapies, nasogastric intubation, medications, and surgical excisions. Nursing care for clients with disorders of the upper digestive tract includes performing a thorough history and physical examination, monitoring intake and output, inserting a nasogastric tube when prescribed, administering feedings through gastric tubes, monitoring vital signs and bowel sounds, preparing the client for diagnostic testing, and teaching the client and family about the disorder and its management.

KEY TERMS

Anorexia	Hiatal hernia
Diverticulum	(diaphragmatic hernia)
Dumping syndrome	Jejunostomy
Dyspepsia	Nasoenteric intubation
Esophagitis	Nasogastric intubation
Fundoplication	Odynophagia
Gastrectomy	Orogastric intubation
Gastric decompression	Peptic ulcer disease
Gastritis	Percutaneous endoscopic
Gastroesophageal reflux	gastrostomy (PEG)
Gastrostomy	Pyrosis

■ Case Studies

1. Mrs. Andrews, age 78, is admitted to the hospital with an unexplained weight loss of 10 lb in the last month. The nurse is preparing to obtain the client's history and perform a physical examination.

2. Mr. Bordman, age 39, visits the clinic complaining of epigastric pain on a daily basis. Nursing history reveals that the client is a traveling salesman who smokes two packs of cigarettes daily, eats "fast food" (usually in his car), and drinks two cocktails at the end of the day.

■ Lippincott Williams & Wilkins Multimedia Resources

Gastrointestinal Pathology Plus, CD-ROM (1999)
Enteral Feeding, video (1997)

■ Internet Resources

GERD/Hiatal Hernia:
www.niddk.nih.gov/health/digest/pubs/heartbrn/heartbrn.htm
H. Pylori:
www.niddk.nih.gov/health/digest/pubs/hpylori/hpylori.htm
Peptic Ulcer:
www.hlm.hih.gov/medlineplus/pepticulcer.html

CHAPTER 53

Caring for Clients With Disorders of the Lower Gastrointestinal Tract

CHAPTER OVERVIEW

The lower gastrointestinal (GI) tract in the human body consists of the small intestine from the duodenum to the anus. Disorders of the lower GI tract often affect the absorption of nutrients, water, and electrolytes; the movement of feces toward the anus; and the elimination of dietary wastes. These disorders include constipation, diarrhea, irritable and inflammatory bowel syndrome, Crohn's disease, ulcerative colitis, appendicitis, peritonitis, intestinal obstructions, diverticular disorders, hernias, cancers of the colon and rectum, hemorrhoids, and anorectal disorders. Nursing care of clients with disorders of the lower GI tract includes taking a thorough history and physical examination, monitoring symptoms and nutritional intake and output, administering prescribed medications, providing preoperative and postoperative care, teaching the client and family about the disorder, and offering referrals to support groups or home care services.

KEY TERMS

Abdominoperineal	Herniorrhaphy
Appendectomy	Inflammatory bowel disease
Appendicitis	Irritable bowel syndrome
Colectomy	Intussusception
Crohn's disease	Paralytic ileus
Diverticula	Peritonitis
Diverticulitis	Pilonidal sinus
Diverticulosis	Segmental resection
Encopresis	Short bowel syndrome
Fissure	Skip lesions
Fistula	Spastic colon
Fistulectomy	Tenesmus
Fistulotomy	Toxic megacolon
Hemorrhoidectomy	Ulcerative colitis
Hemorrhoids	Ulcerative proctitis
Hernia	Volvulus
Hernioplasty	

■ Case Studies

1. A nurse on a medical unit is notified by the admitting department that a client is to be admitted. The client, Mrs. Chandler, age 35, is to be admitted as a result of complications due to ulcerative colitis.

2. A nurse is caring for Mrs. Monty, age 82, who is bedridden following a total hip replacement. When the nurse assists the client off a bedpan, the nurse observes blood on the toilet tissue.

3. The nurse is caring for Mr. Zellman, age 75, who is scheduled for insertion of a nasogastric tube for decompression.

■ Lippincott Williams & Wilkins Multimedia Resources

Gastrointestinal Pathology Plus, CD-ROM (1999)

■ Internet Resources

Diverticulitis: http://gutfeelings.com
Crohn's Disease: www.access.admin.mcmaster.ca/csd/resources/colitis.html
Hemorrhoids: www.niddk.nih.gov/health/digest/pubs/hems/hemords.htm

CHAPTER 54

Caring for Clients With an Ileostomy or Colostomy

CHAPTER OVERVIEW

The most common intestinal ostomies are the ileostomy, which is an opening from the distal small intestine, and the colostomy, which is an opening from the colon. Fecal material exits through a stoma. For a conventional ileostomy, the entire colon and rectum are removed. A temporary or permanent colostomy may be created in the ascending, transverse, descending, or sigmoid area of the colon. Physicians may prescribe colostomy irrigations. Nursing care for clients who need ostomies includes doing a thorough history and physical examination, performing preoperative and postoperative teaching and preparation, monitoring intake and output and vital signs, administering prescribed medications or intravenous fluids, preventing injury, teaching about diet and health, providing stoma care and irrigation and skin care, counseling regarding sexual concerns, and maintaining adequate tissue perfusion.

■ Key Terms

Abdominoperineal resection
Appliance
Colostomy
Continent ileostomy (Kock pouch)
Conventional ileostomy
Double-barrel colostomy
Effluent
Enterostomal therapist

Ileoanal reservoir (anastomosis)
Ileostomy
Loop colostomy
Ostomate
Ostomy
Segmental resection
Single-barrel colostomy
Stoma

■ Case Studies

1. A nurse is caring for two clients: Ms. Lipton, age 20, with an ileostomy, and Mr. Rhodes, age 60, with a colostomy.

2. A nurse is caring for Mr. Sax, age 55, who has recently undergone surgery for an ileostomy. He tells the nurse, "I'm sure getting tired of emptying this bag so often every day. I think I'll just decrease my fluid intake so I don't have to change the bag so often."

3. A nurse is caring for Mrs. Wiles, age 55, who has a permanent colostomy. The client tells the nurse, "I sure seem to have a lot of 'gas' lately. Do you think something is wrong?"

■ Lippincott Williams & Wilkins Multimedia Resources

Gastrointestinal Pathology Plus, CD-ROM (1999)

■ Internet Resources

British Colostomy Support and Information: www.bcass.org.uk/
Ileostomy: www.niddk.nigh.gov/health/digest/ summary/iostomy/iostomy.htm
United Ostomy Association: www.uoa.org/ uoa-9.html
Ostomy: www.ostomy.fsnet.co.uk/

CHAPTER 55

Caring for Clients With Disorders of the Liver, Gallbladder, and Pancreas

CHAPTER OVERVIEW

When there are disorders of the liver, gallbladder, or pancreas, digestion of foods is affected. Liver disorders include jaundice, cirrhosis, esophageal varices, hepatitis, and tumors. Gallbladder disorders include cholelithiasis and cholecystitis. Pancreatic disorders include pancreatitis and cancer of the pancreas. Nursing care of clients with these disorders includes a thorough history and physical examination; pre- and postoperative teaching and care; administration of prescribed medications; prevention of injury; monitoring of intake and output; nutritional health teaching; administration of enteral feedings such as TPN; assistance with diagnostic testing and biopsies; following universal precautions to prevent infections; pain control; skin integrity; and care of T-tubes. The nurse is also responsible for referrals to support groups or home health care services.

KEY TERMS

Alpha-fetoprotein
Ascites
Biliary colic
Caput medusae
Cholecystitis
Choledocholithiasis
Cholelithiasis
Cirrhosis
Cullen's sign
Esophageal varices
Fetor hepaticus
Hepatic lobectomy
Hepatitis
Hepatorenal syndrome
Injection sclerotherapy

Laparoscopic
    cholecystectomy
Lithotripsy
Open cholecystectomy
Pancreatectomy
    (partial, total)
Pancreatitis
Portal hypertension
Radical pancreatico-
    ducidenectomy
(Whipple procedure)
Steatorrhea
T-tube
Turner's sign

■ Case Studies

1. Mr. Demming, age 58, visits the clinic and complains of jaundice. The nurse observes that the client's skin appears yellow.

2. The nurse is talking to Carol, age 16, who has indicated a desire to become a nurse. During the conversation Carol tells the nurse, "Although I am considering nursing as a career, I am afraid I might catch something, like hepatitis B or HIV."

3. The nurse is caring for two clients: Mrs. Nolan, age 58, scheduled for a laparoscopic cholecystectomy, and Mr. Brown, age 65, scheduled for an open cholecystectomy.

■ Lippincott Williams & Wilkins Multimedia Resources

Gastointestinal Pathology Plus, CD-ROM (1999)

■ Internet Resources

Hepatitis C: www.hna.ffh.vic.gove.au/phb/hprot/idci/hepC.html
Hepatitis C: www.hepatiti-c.de
Liver Transplant: www.gastro.com/liverpg/tranfaqs.htm
Pancreatitis: www.niddk.nih.gov/health/digest/pubs/pancreas/pancreas.htm
Pancreatitis: www.gastro.org/public/pancreatitis.html

CHAPTER 56

Introduction to the Endocrine System

CHAPTER OVERVIEW

The major functions of the endocrine system include metabolism, growth, fluid and electrolyte balance, reproductive processes, and sleep-wake cycles. Endocrine glands secrete hormones directly into the bloodstream. These hormones accelerate or slow physiologic processes. The hypothalamus regulates the pituitary gland. Other endocrine glands include the thyroid, parathyroids, thymus, pineal gland, adrenal glands, pancreas, ovaries, and testes. General nursing care for clients suspected of having disorders of the endocrine system includes a thorough history (including diet and medications), a physical examination (including mental status examination), allergies (especially iodine), height and weight measurements, preparing the client for and assisting with diagnostic testing and laboratory studies, and client and family teaching related to diet, medications, and care following diagnostic testing.

KEY TERMS

Adenohypophysis	nuclear scan
Adrenal cortex	Ovaries
Adrenal glands	Oxytocin
Adrenal medulla	Pancreas
Adrenocorticotropic	Parathormone
hormone	Parathyroid glands
Antidiuretic hormone	Pineal gland
Calcitonin	Pituitary gland
Corticosteroids	Progesterone
Estrogen	Prolactin
Feedback loop	Radionuclide
Follicle-stimulating	Nuclear scan
hormone	Somatotropin
Glucagon	Testes
Glycogenolysis	Testosterone
Hormones	Tetraiodothyronine
Hypophysis	Thymosin
Hypothalamus	Thymus gland
Insulin	Thyroid gland
Islets of Langerhans	Thyroid-stimulating hormone
Luteinizing hormone	Triiodothyronine
Melatonin	
Neurohypophysis	

■ Case Studies

1. The nurse is planning a presentation about the endocrine system to a group of high school students. The nurse plans to begin the discussion with the pituitary gland.

2. The nurse is planning a presentation to a group of adult women about the endocrine system and the feedback loop of the system.

■ Lippincott Williams & Wilkins Multimedia Resources

Performing Head-to-Toe Assessment, video (2000)

■ Internet Resource

Endocrine System: www.endocrineweb.com

CHAPTER 57

Caring for Clients With Disorders of the Endocrine System

CHAPTER OVERVIEW

For clients with a disorder of an endocrine gland, the nurse should pay particular attention to the effects of the disorder on other endocrine glands. Disorders of the endocrine system include acromegaly, panhypopituitarism, diabetes insipidus, hyperthyroidism, hypothyroidism, thyroid tumors, goiters, thyroiditis, hyperparathyroidism, Addison's disease, pheochromocytoma, Cushing's syndrome, hyperaldosteronism, and disorders of the ovaries and testes. Nursing care of clients diagnosed with disorders of the endocrine system includes thorough history and physical examination, monitoring intake and output, counseling regarding sexual concerns, monitoring level of consciousness and sleep-wake cycles, vital sign assessments, administration of prescribed medications, preoperative and postoperative care, assisting with diagnostic testing, and client and family teaching related to the disorder, medications, postoperative care, and referral to support groups or home care services.

KEY TERMS

Acromegaly	Hypophysectomy
Addisonian crisis	Hypothyroidism
Adrenal insufficiency	Myxedema
Adrenalectomy	Pheochromocytoma
Carpopedal spasm	Simmonds' disease
Chvostek's sign	Syndrome of inappropriate
Cushingoid syndrome	antidiuretic hormone
Diabetes insipidus	secretion
Goiter	Tetany
Hyperparathyroidism	Thyroiditis
Hyperplasia	Thyrotoxic crisis
Hyperthyroidism	Trousseau's sign
Hypoparathyroidism	

■ Case Studies

1. The nurse is caring for Mrs. Swanson, age 60, following a bilateral adrenalectomy. The client is scheduled to receive fludrocortisone orally. The charge nurse asks the staff members for suggestions on how to be sure the client receives her medications in a timely manner.

2. The nurse is caring for Mr. Wiles, age 55, who had a thyroidectomy this morning. It is now 8:00 PM and the client is complaining of difficulty in swallowing clear liquids and a "fullness in her throat." There is no drainage on the client's surgical dressing. Blood pressure is 120/80. Pulse is 124 beats per minute.

■ Lippincott Williams & Wilkins Multimedia Resources

Performing Head-to-Toe Assessment, video (2000)

■ Internet Resource

Endocrine System: www.nlm.nih.gov/medlineplus/endocrinesystemhormones.html

CHAPTER 58

Caring for Clients With Diabetes Mellitus

CHAPTER OVERVIEW

The two major groups of diabetes mellitus include type I diabetes mellitus, which typically occurs in juveniles and is also called insulin-dependent diabetes mellitus (IDDM), and type II diabetes mellitus, which typically occurs in adulthood and is also called non-insulin-dependent diabetes mellitus (NIDDM). Although there is no known cause, it is believed that a combination of factors predisposes an individual to diabetes mellitus. Excess glucose in the blood leads to hyperglycemia. Symptoms of diabetes mellitus include excessive urination (polyuria), excessive thirst (polydipsia), increased hunger with weight loss, ketones in the urine (ketonuria), ketoacidosis with Kussmaul respirations, and, potentially, diabetic coma. Diagnostic testing for diabetes mellitus includes testing for ketones in the urine and performing a fasting blood glucose, a postprandial glucose, and an oral glucose tolerance test. Medical management includes a special diet, exercise, weight control, insulin or an oral diabetic agent, and counseling regarding lifestyle changes. Nursing care for clients with diabetes includes a obtaining a thorough history, physical examination, and diet history; assisting with diagnostic testing; instructing the client about insulin administration, diet, and exercise; providing client and family teaching related to potential complications; monitoring the client for complications (e.g., ketoacidosis or coma); monitoring vital signs and blood glucose levels; and assisting with skin and foot care.

KEY TERMS

Diabetes mellitus	Ketonemia
Diabetic coma	Ketones
Diabetic ketoacidosis	Kussmaul respirations
Fasting blood glucose	Lipoatrophy
Glycosuria	Lipolysis
Glycosylated hemoglobin	Metabolic syndrome
Hyperglycemia	Oral glucose tolerance test
Hyperinsulinism	Polydipsia
Hyperosmolar hyperglycemic nonketotic syndrome	Polyphagia
	Polyuria
Hypoglycemia	Postprandial glucose
Insulin independence	Renal threshold
Ketoacidosis	

■ Case Studies

1. Mrs. Wilton, age 55, has recently been diagnosed with NIDDM, and she visits the clinic for a routine examination. The client tells the nurse, "I just can't seem to stay on that diet the doctor put me on. I love to bake and I enjoy my 'sweets' even though I know I'm not supposed to have them."

2. The nurse is planning to instruct Julie, age 16, about her diabetes mellitus. The primary focus of this teaching session includes signs and symptoms of hypoglycemia and hyperglycemia.

3. The nurse is caring for Mark, age 15, diagnosed with type I diabetes. The physician has ordered a daily injection of NPH insulin 40 U, and regular insulin 20 U. The nurse is planning to instruct Mark how to draw up the insulin into a single syringe.

■ Lippincott Williams & Wilkins Multimedia Resources

Performing Head-to-Toe Assessment, video (2000)

■ Internet Resources

American Diabetes Association: www.diabetes.org
Diabetes Public Health Resources: www.cdc.gov/diabetes
Juvenile Diabetes: www.jdf.org
National Institute of Diabetes & Digestive & Kidney Disease: www.niddk.nih.gov

Caring for Clients With Disorders of Pelvic Reproductive Structures

CHAPTER OVERVIEW

The external structures of the female reproductive system consist of the breasts, the vaginal orifice, the labia majora, the labia minora, and the clitoris. The internal structures include the uterus, two ovaries, two fallopian tubes, and the vagina. Monthly ovulation is the release of ova for fertilization by the sperm, resulting in pregnancy. If no pregnancy results, menstruation occurs. During menstruation, the lining of the uterus is sloughed off, usually beginning about 2 weeks after ovulation. During a gynecologic examination, various diagnostic tests can be performed. These tests include PAP smear, cervical biopsy, endometrial smears and biopsies, and dilatation and curettage. Other tests include endoscopic examinations, hysterosalpingogram, abdominal ultrasonography, and laboratory tests. Disorders of the female reproductive system include menstrual disorders; menopause; infectious and inflammatory disorders, such as vaginitis and pelvic inflammatory disease; structural abnormalities, such as endometriosis, fistulas, or pelvic organ prolapse; tumors of the reproductive system, such as leiomyomas; cysts; and cervical, endometrial, vaginal, vulvar, and ovarian cancers. Nursing care for clients diagnosed with female reproductive structure disorders includes obtaining a thorough health history and physical examination, including a gynecologic examination; assisting with diagnostic testing and laboratory studies; providing preoperative and postoperative teaching and care; monitoring vital signs; administering prescribed medications; promoting pain management; maintaining skin integrity; administering chemotherapy; teaching the client and family about the disorder; and referring the client to support groups or home health care services.

KEY TERMS

Abortion	Mammography
Amenorrhea	Menarche
Artificial insemination	Menopause
Carcinoma in situ	Menorrhagia
Cervicitis	Menstrual diary
Conization	Menstruation
Cystocele	Menstruation
Dysmenorrhea	Metrorrhagia
Dyspareunia	Oligomenorrhea
Endometriosis	Oophorectomy
Fertilization	Ova
Fibroid tumor	Ovulation
Fistula	Pelvic inflammatory
Gametes	disease
Gynecologic examination	Premenstrual syndrome
Hormone replacement	Puberty
therapy	Rectocele
Hysterectomy	Salpingectomy
Implantation	Sterility
Kegel's exercises	Toxic shock syndrome
Libido	Vaginitis

■ Case Studies

1. A newly married couple visits the clinic. The young woman tells the nurse that just before her menstrual cycle, she is irritable, feels "bloated," and craves sugary foods. The client's husband tells the nurse, "I think it's all in her head."

2. The nurse is caring for Ms. Lusker, age 17, who has been diagnosed with possible premenstrual syndrome. The nurse plans to instruct the client about keeping a menstrual diary for 2 months and then returning to the clinic.

3. The nurse is planning a presentation to a group of adult women on the topic of "Female Reproductive Cancers."

4. The nurse is caring for Mrs. Dorchett, age 52, who has just been diagnosed as menopausal.

■ Lippincott Williams & Wilkins Multimedia Resources

Clinical Gynecological Endocrinology and Infertility, Sixth Edition, CD-ROM (2001)
GyneE, CD-ROM (1999)
Vaginal Surgery Video Series, video (1996)

■ Internet Resources

Gynecologic Diseases: www.womenshealth.org
Infertility: www.ihr.com/infertility

CHAPTER 60

Caring for Clients With Breast Disorders

CHAPTER OVERVIEW

The female breasts contain the mammary glands, which are a network of ducts that carry milk to the nipple following pregnancy and delivery of a newborn. The axillary lymph nodes and the internal mammary lymph nodes drain the breasts. Regular breast self-examination on a monthly basis is recommended for all women. Mammography is recommended for women over the age of 40. Mammography should be done every 1 to 2 years until the age of 50, when it should be performed annually. Breast biopsy may be done to determine if a breast lesion is malignant. Breast disorders include infectious and inflammatory breast disorders, such as mastitis or abscess. Fibrocystic breast disease with benign lesions may be chronic or acute. Malignant breast disorders include malignant tumors or tumors with metastases. Treatment depends on the stage of the disease and may include surgical removal of the tumor or breast, radiation, and chemotherapy. Cosmetic breast procedures include breast reconstruction, reduction mammoplasty, breast lift, and breast augmentation. Nursing care for clients with breast disorders includes obtaining a thorough history and physical examination, assisting with diagnostic testing, teaching related to breast self-examination and diagnostic testing, performing preoperative and postoperative care, managing pain, checking vital signs, changing surgical dressing, and providing client and family health teaching.

KEY TERMS

Breast abscess	Mastalgia
Breast cancer	Mastitis
Breast reconstruction	Mastopexy
Breast self-examination	Modified radical mastectomy
Clinical breast examination	Partial (or segmental)
Fibroadenoma	mastectomy
Fibrocystic breast disease	Reduction mammoplasty
Lumpectomy	Sentinel lymph node
Lymphedema	mapping/biopsy
Mammography	Simple (or total) mastectomy
Mammoplasty	Subcutaneous mastectomy

■ Case Studies

1. The nurse is caring for the following clients: Mrs. Bellow, age 35, diagnosed with chronic fibrocystic breast disease; Mrs. Kindred, age 50, diagnosed with fibroadenoma; and Mrs. Jules, age 66, diagnosed with a malignant breast tumor.

2. The nurse is planning a presentation to a group of young women on the topic of breast cancer prevention.

3. The nurse is caring for the following clients: Mrs. Packer, age 56, who had a radical mastectomy and desires breast reconstruction surgery; Mrs. Trowly, age 26, who desires breast augmentation; and Ms. Penn, age 22, who desires breast reduction surgery.

■ Lippincott Williams & Wilkins Multimedia Resources

Atlas of Breast Pathology, CD-ROM (1997)
The Breast, CD-ROM (1998)

■ Internet Resources

Breast Cancer: www.nabco.org
Fibrocystic Breast Disease: www.healthy.net/library/ books/lark/fcbdises.html

CHAPTER 61

Caring for Clients With Disorders of the Male Reproductive System

CHAPTER OVERVIEW

In the male, the lower urinary tract and the reproductive system structures are so closely related that disorders often affect both systems. The external male genitalia consist of the penis and the scrotum. The testes lie within the scrotum and are responsible for spermatogenesis and the secretion of testosterone. Internal genitalia include the epididymides, vas deferens, seminal vesicles, prostate gland, and bulbourethral glands. Structural abnormalities include cryptorchidism (undescended testes), torsion of the spermatic cord, phimosis and paraphimosis, hydrocele, spermatocele, and varicocele. Infectious or inflammatory disorders include prostatitis, epididymitis, and orchitis. Erection disorders include priapism and impotence. Benign prostatic hyperplasia (BPH) occurs as men age. Malignancies include cancer of the prostate, cancer of the testes, and cancer of the penis. A vasectomy results in sterilization, and reversal of a vasectomy attempts to restore sperm production. Nursing care for male clients with reproductive disorders includes obtaining a thorough history and physical examination, assisting with diagnostic testing, providing preoperative and postoperative care, counseling regarding sexuality issues, monitoring intake and output and vital signs, assisting the client in maintaining bladder control, administering medications, providing client and family health teaching, and referring the client to home care or support groups.

■ Case Studies

1. A nurse is caring for two clients: Mr. Silvers, age 60, who will undergo a TURP, and Mr. Cone, age 23, who will undergo a radical inguinal orchiectomy with retroperitoneal lymph node dissection.

2. A nurse is leading a team conference to plan the care for Mr. Rogers, age 58, who is scheduled for a suprapubic prostatectomy in the morning.

3. A nurse is planning a presentation to a group of males on the topic of prostate hypertrophy and testicular cancer.

■ Internet Resources

BPH: www.pslgroup.com/enlargprost.htm
Erectile Dysfunction: www.impotence.org
Prostate Cancer: www.4npcc.org
Testicular Cancer: www.acor.org/diseases/TC

KEY TERMS

Benign prostatic hyperplasia	Prostatectomy
Cryptorchidism	Prostatic specific antigen
Digital rectal	Retrograde ejaculation
Ejaculation	Semen
Epididymitis	Spermatogenesis
Impotence	Testicular self-examination
Orchiectomy	Transillumination
Orchitis	Tumor markers
Orchiopexy	Vasectomy

CHAPTER 62

Caring for Clients With Sexually Transmitted Diseases

CHAPTER OVERVIEW

Sexually transmitted diseases, which are also termed venereal diseases, are infections that are spread through sexual activity. Besides AIDS, the five most common sexually transmitted diseases include *Chlamydia*, gonorrhea, syphilis, genital herpes, and genital warts. The most common and fastest spreading disease is *Chlamydia*. Some factors that contribute to the high incidence of venereal disease include ignorance of how the diseases are spread; casual sexual contact; multiple partners; failure to use contraceptive techniques, such as condoms; and mutation and resistance of the organisms to antimicrobial therapy. Nursing care for clients experiencing a sexually transmitted disease includes obtaining an accurate and thorough history and physical examination, using universal blood and bodily fluid precautions, assisting with specimen collection and treatment, administering prescribed medications, providing health teaching related to the spread of the disease and prevention techniques (e.g., condoms), monitoring symptoms of disease progression, preparing the client for diagnostic testing, assisting with laser or cryosurgery, and teaching the client and family about the disease.

KEY TERMS

Autoinoculation	Granuloma inguinale
Chancre	Herpes simplex virus
Chancroid	Human papilloma virus
Charcot's joints	Lymphogranuloma venereum
Chlamydia	Neuropathic joint disease
Condyloma	Syphilis
Genital herpes	Tabes dorsalis
Gonorrhea	Venereal diseases

■ Case Studies

1. The nurse is caring for a client who tells the nurse, "I don't know who else to tell this to. My boyfriend thinks he's the only one; however, I'm also having sex with his friend. This has been going on for a few weeks. I never use any kind of protection."

2. The nurse is caring for a male client who tells the nurse, "I've never used a condom before. What do I need to know about using a condom?"

■ Internet Resources

Sexually Transmitted Infection Facts:
    www.plannedparenthood.org/sti
STD Prevention:
    www.cdc.gov/nchstp/dstd/dstdp.html

CHAPTER 63

Introduction to the Urinary Tract

CHAPTER OVERVIEW

The upper urinary tract is composed of the kidneys, ureters, and renal pelves, while the lower urinary tract is composed of the bladder, urethra, and pelvic floor muscles. The kidneys excrete excess water and wastes; maintain the acid-base of the body; produce the enzyme renin, which raises the blood pressure; and produce the hormone erythropoietin, which regulates blood cell production. Twenty five percent of the total cardiac output is received by the kidneys. Diagnostic tests for urinary tract disorders include radiography, ultrasonography, computed tomography (CT) scan, magnetic resonance imaging, angiography, cystoscopy, intravenous pyelogram and retrograde pyelogram, biopsy, cystogram, and voiding cystourethrogram. Laboratory tests include urinalysis, urine culture and sensitivity, 24-hour urine collection, urine-specific gravity, urine protein, creatinine clearance test, and blood chemistries. General nursing care for clients with urinary tract disorders includes obtaining a thorough history and physical examination, explaining and preparing the client for diagnostic testing and laboratory studies, assisting with specimen collection, counseling about nutrition and diet, administering prescribed medications, carefully observing and monitoring after diagnostic testing, teaching the client and family about the disorder, and referring to support groups or home care services.

KEY TERMS

Blood urea nitrogen	Renal arteriogram
Creatinine	Retrograde pyelogram
Creatinine clearance test	Ultrasonography
Cystogram	Urinalysis
Cystometrogram	Urine protein test
Cystoscope	Urine specific gravity
Cystoscopy	Urodynamic studies
Excretory urogram	Uroflowmetry
intravenous pyelogram	Urography
Post void residual	Voiding cystourethrogram

■ Case Studies

1. The nurse is caring for Mr. Hook, age 35, who is scheduled for a cystoscopy and a retrograde pyelogram. The client appears very nervous. He says to the nurse, "I am really scared about all of these tests. What are they for? How long do I have to be here? When will I know the results? Can my wife be with me? Is this going to hurt?"

2. The nurse is caring for Ms. Maple, age 40. She is scheduled for culture and sensitivity, an ultrasound, a renal angiogram, a cystoscopy, and a retrograde pyelogram.

■ Lippincott Williams & Wilkins Multimedia Resources

Performing Head-to-Toe Assessment, video (2000)

■ Internet Resource

Endocrine System: www.endocrineweb.com

CHAPTER 64

Caring for Clients With Disorders of the Kidneys and Ureters

CHAPTER OVERVIEW

The most common urologic disorders are infectious and inflammatory conditions, which can lead to acute or chronic renal failure. These conditions include pyelonephritis (a bacterial infection of the kidney), acute or chronic glomerulonephritis, congenital kidney disorders (e.g., polycystic kidneys), and obstructive disorders, such as kidney and ureteral stones, ureteral strictures, kidney tumors, and acute or chronic renal failure. Depending on the disorder, these clients may need treatment with lithotripsy or dialysis. Nursing care for clients with these disorders includes obtaining a comprehensive history and thorough physical examination, providing preoperative and postoperative nursing care, administering prescribed medications, providing pain control, assisting with specimen collection and diagnostic testing, monitoring intake and output, encouraging or limiting fluid intake, reviewing laboratory studies, counseling about nutrition and diet, assisting with therapies such as dialysis, teaching the client and family about the disorder, and referring to support groups or home care services.

KEY TERMS

Acute renal failure	Hematuria
Acute tubular necrosis	Hemodialysis
Anasarca	Hydronephrosis
Anuria	Nephrectomy
Arteriovenous fistula	Nephrolithiasis
Arteriovenous graft	Nephrostomy tube
Azotemia	Nocturia
Bruit	Oliguria
Calciuria	Osteodystrophy
Calculus	Periorbital edema
Casts	Peritoneal dialysis
Chronic renal failure	Pyelonephritis
Colic	Pyeloplasty
Dialysate	Pyuria
Dialysis	Thrill
Dialyzer	Uremia
Disequilibrium syndrome	Uremic frost
End-stage renal disease	Ureteral stent
Extracorporeal shock	Ureterolithiasis
wave lithotripsy	Ureteroplasty
Glomerulonephritis	Urolithiasis

■ Case Studies

1. The nurse is caring for Mr. Abbott, age 40, who is being treated for ureteral stones. The client tells the nurse that he is experiencing severe pain. As the nurse prepares to obtain the client's prescribed pain medication, another nurse on the unit tells her, "Oh, you're caring for Mr. Abbott? He has a really low pain tolerance."

2. The nurse is caring for Mrs. Wallace, who had a left nephrectomy earlier in the day. The client tells the nurse, "I'm having a lot of discomfort when I have to cough, deep breathe, or change positions."

3. If you had chronic renal failure and must decide to have either hemodialysis or peritoneal dialysis when end-stage disease develops, explain which choice you would make and the reasons for the choice.

■ Lippincott Williams & Wilkins Multimedia Resources

Performing Head-to-Toe Assessment, video (2000)

■ Internet Resource

Urinary Diseases: www.nih.gov/medlineplus/kidneysandurinarysystem.html

CHAPTER 65

Caring for Clients With Disorders of the Bladder and Urethra

CHAPTER OVERVIEW

Although many disorders of the bladder and urethra are treated on an outpatient basis, the more serious disorders require hospitalization. Voiding dysfunctions include urinary retention and urinary incontinence. Urinary retention requires catheterization to alleviate the problem. Urinary incontinence is a major health concern and can affect the client's quality of life. Treatment is aimed at correcting the problem. Infectious and inflammatory disorders include cystitis and urethritis. Obstructive disorders include bladder stones and urethral strictures. Malignant tumors of the bladder may require surgical removal of the bladder. Various types of injuries can result in trauma to the bladder or urethra and may require surgical treatment. Nursing care of clients with bladder or urethral disorders includes obtaining a thorough history and physical examination, assisting with laboratory specimens and diagnostic testing, assisting the client with a bladder rehabilitation program, monitoring intake and output, performing preoperative and postoperative care and skin care, providing fluid and nutrition counseling, administering prescribed medications, teaching the client and family about the disorder, and providing referrals to support groups or home health services.

KEY TERMS

Cystectomy	Neurogenic bladder
Cystitis	Residual urine
Cystostomy	Retention
Diverticulum	Stricture
Fulguration	Urethritis
Incontinence	Urethroplasty
Interstitial cystitis	Urinary diversion
Litholapaxy	Urosepsis

■ Case Studies

1. The nurse is caring for a client who has experienced chronic bladder infections (cystitis). The physician has told the client that she should have a cystoscopy and retrograde pyelogram. The client asks the nurse, "Why do I need to have these tests? When I was here before with the same problems, he just gave me a prescription for some medicine."

2. The nurse is caring for a client with interstitial cystitis who appears very distraught.

3. The nurse is caring for a client who has just undergone a ureterosigmoidostomy. The nurse plans to instruct the client about long-term management and care.

■ Lippincott Williams & Wilkins Multimedia Resources

Performing Head-to-Toe Assessment, video (2000)

■ Internet Resources

Incontinence: www.ahcpr.gov/clinic/uiovervw.htm
Interstitial Cystitis: www.ichelp.com
Non-gonorrheal Urethritis: www.ashastd.org/stdfaqs/ngu.html
Urinary Tract Infection: www.niddk.nih.gov/health/urolog/pubs/utiadult/utiadult.htm

CHAPTER 66

Introduction to the Musculoskeletal System

CHAPTER OVERVIEW

This chapter describes the major structures of the musculoskeletal system. Bones can be either cancellous bone or spongy bone, cortical bone, or dense, compact bone. Skeletal muscles are voluntary muscles that are controlled by impulses that travel from efferent nerves of the brain and spinal cord. A joint is a junction between two or more bones. Tendons are cordlike structures that attach muscles to the periosteum. A bursa is a small, fluid-filled sac filled with synovial fluid. Diagnostic tests include radiography, computed tomography, magnetic resonance imaging, arthroscopy, synovial fluid analysis, bone scans, biopsies, and 24-hour urine tests for uric acid levels. General nursing care for clients experiencing musculoskeletal disorders includes a thorough history and physical examination; assisting with diagnostic and laboratory testing; determining circulatory status following an injury; pain and anxiety management; pre-and postoperative care; administering prescribed medications; teaching about safety and rest; client and family health teaching related to the disorder; and referring the client to support groups or home care services.

KEY TERMS

Arthrocentesis	Joint
Arthrogram	Ligament
Arthroscopy	Ossification
Bone scan	Osteoblasts
Bursa	Osteocytes
Calcification	Periosteum
Cancellous bone	Red bone marrow
Cartilage	Resorption
Cortical bone	Skeletal muscles
Diaphyses	Tendon
Epiphyses	Yellow bone marrow

■ Case Studies

1. The nurse is working in a long-term care setting when one of the clients falls while walking in the hallway.

2. The nurse is caring for Mr. Patman, age 55, who suffered a fractured arm when he fell from a ladder.

■ Lippincott Williams & Wilkins Multimedia Resources

Achland's Video Atlas of Human Anatomy, video (2000)
Performing Head-To-Toe Assessment, video (2000)

■ Internet Resources

Musculoskeletal Graphics: www.eduserv.hscer. washington.edu/hubio553/atlas

Caring for Clients With Orthopedic and Connective Tissue Disorders

CHAPTER OVERVIEW

Disorders that affect the musculoskeletal system can affect the individual's ability to perform activities of daily living. Musculoskeletal disorders include sprains, dislocations, fractures, rheumatoid arthritis, degenerative joint disease, gout, bursitis, ankylosing spondylitis, Lyme disease, lupus erythematosus, back pain, osteoporosis, bone tumors, and amputations. Nursing care for clients with musculoskeletal disorders includes obtaining a thorough history and physical examination, assisting with diagnostic and laboratory testing, determining circulatory status following an injury, managing pain and anxiety, providing preoperative and postoperative care, assessing casts, assessing mobility, assessing the client's ability to carry out activities of daily living, administering prescribed medications, teaching about safety and rest, giving medication, counseling the client on diet and nutrition, providing client and family health teaching related to the disorder, and referring the client to support groups or home care services.

KEY TERMS

Ankylosing spondylitis	Hammertoe
Ankylosis	Hyperuricemia
Arthritis	Internal fixation
Arthrodesis	Involucrum
Arthroplasty	Lupus erythematosus
Avascular necrosis	Lyme disease
Avulsion fracture	Open reduction
Bouchard's nodes	Osseous ankylosis
Bursitis	Osteomalacia
Callus	Osteomyelitis
Carpal tunnel syndrome	Osteoporosis
Cast	Osteotomy
Closed reduction	Paget's disease
Compartment syndrome	Palsy
Contusion	Pannus
Degenerative joint disease	Rheumatoid arthritis
Dislocation	Sequestrum
Ecchymosis	Sprain
Epicondylitis	Strain
External fixation	Subluxation
Fasciotomy	Synovectomy
Fibrous ankylosis	Synovitis
Fracture	Tophi
Gout	Traction
Heberden's nodes	Volkmann's contracture

■ Case Studies

1. The nurse is caring for Mr. White, age 65, who had a total hip replacement 3 days ago. The client tells the nurse he needs to use the bedpan to have a bowel movement.

2. The nurse is caring for Mrs. Wonder, age 87, following an AK amputation 2 hours ago. The nurse observes that the client's stump dressing is saturated with blood.

■ Lippincott Williams & Wilkins Multimedia Resources

Performing Head-to-Toe Assessment, video (2000)

■ Internet Resources

Degenerative Joint Disease:
    www.wokc2.com/degenjoint.htm
Ergonomics: www.cdc.gov/niosh/ergosci1.html
Musculoskeletal Diseases:
    www.mic.ki.se/Diseases/c5.html
Rheumatoid Arthritis:
    www.rheumatology.org.nz/nz080000.htm

CHAPTER 68

Introduction to the Integumentary System

CHAPTER OVERVIEW

The skin is the largest organ of the body, and it is divided into two layers: the epidermis, or outer layer, and the dermis, or inner layer. Skin color is determined by the amount of melanin. The skin has four major functions: protection, temperature regulation, sensory processing, and chemical synthesis. Hair originates from the hair follicles within the dermis. Sebaceous glands are connected to the hair follicles and secrete sebum. Sweat glands include both eccrine glands and apocrine glands. Nails are layers of hard keratin that have a protective function. General nursing care for clients with disorders of the integumentary system includes obtaining a thorough history and physical examination; assisting with diagnostic and laboratory testing; determining circulatory status following an injury; preventing, staging, and treating pressure sores; providing pain and anxiety management; providing preoperative and postoperative care; administering prescribed medications and treatments; teaching about safety and rest; giving medication, diet, and nutrition counseling; teaching the client and family about the disorder and potential lifestyle changes; and referring the client to support groups or home care services.

KEY TERMS

Apocrine glands
Debridement
Dermis
Eccrine glands
Epidermis
Integument
Keratin
Melanin
Pheromones

Pressure sores
Sebaceous glands
Sebum
Shearing
Skin tear
Stratum corneum
Subcutaneous tissue
Sweat glands

■ Case Study

1. The nurse is caring for Mrs. Vine, age 68, who has developed a rash over her arms and thorax.

■ Lippincott Williams & Wilkins Multimedia Resources

Performing Head-to-Toe Assessment, video (2000)

■ Internet Resources

American Academy of Dermatology: www.aad.org
Dermatology Foundation: www.dermfnd.org

CHAPTER 69

Caring for Clients With Skin, Hair, and Nail Disorders

CHAPTER OVERVIEW

Disorders of the skin, hair, and nails, are common disorders and can affect the client's self-esteem. Dermatitis is a term used to describe inflammation of the skin. Acne vulgaris is an inflammatory disorder that involves the sebaceous glands and hair follicles. Other skin disorders include furuncles (boils), psoriasis, scabies, dermatophytoses, shingles (herpes zoster), and skin cancer. Scalp and hair disorders include seborrhea, seborrheic dermatitis, dandruff, alopecia (baldness), and head lice (pediculosis). Nail disorders include onychomycosis and onychocryptosis. Nursing care for clients with integumentary system disorders includes obtaining a thorough history and physical examination; assisting with diagnostic and laboratory testing; providing pain and anxiety management; providing preoperative and postoperative care; administering prescribed medications and treatments; ensuring safety and rest; providing medication, diet, and nutrition counseling; counseling about hygiene, prevention of transmission (e.g., head lice), and use of sunscreen products; teaching the client and family about the disorder and potential lifestyle changes; and referring to support groups or home care services.

KEY TERMS

Acne vulgaris	Furuncle
Alopecia	Furunculosis
Autograft	Herpes zoster
Carbuncle	Nits
Comedones	Onychocryptosis
Debridement	Onychomycosis
Dermabrasion	Pediculosis
Dermatitis	Podiatrist
Dermatome	Pruritus
Dermatophytes	Psoriasis
Dermatophytoses	Scabies
Epithelialization	Shingles
Erythema	Slit graft

■ Case Studies

1. The nurse is planning a presentation to a group of high school students on the topic of "Healthy Skin, Hair, and Nails."

2. The nurse is caring for two clients: Mr. Bard, age 15, diagnosed with a skin disorder, and Mrs. Little, age 65, diagnosed with a skin disorder.

■ Lippincott Williams & Wilkins Multimedia Resources

Performing Head-to-Toe Assessment, video (2000)

■ Internet Resources

Alopecia: www.alopeciaareata.com
Acne: http://medlib.med.utah.edu/kw/derm/acne
Decubitus Ulcers: www.decubitus.org
Eczema: www.eczema.org
Psoriasis: www.psoriasis.org

Caring for Clients With Burns

CHAPTER OVERVIEW

Burns are a serious, life-threatening injury that may be caused by heat, chemicals, or electricity. Complications from burns may be from fluid loss, fluid shift, or wound infection. Extent of injury can be determined from depth of the burn, amount of tissue affected, and location. The nurse is responsible for assessing burned areas, identifying complications, removing eschar, and treating wounds. Pain control is an essential part of nursing care, as is promoting nutrition and fluid balance.

KEY TERMS

Allograft	Full-thickness graft
Autograft	Heterograft
Closed method	Open method
Epithelialization	Slit graft
Escharotomy	Split-thickness graft
Eschar	

■ Case Studies

1. A client has spilled a cup of hot coffee on his lap, resulting in second-degree burns of his genital area.

2. The nurse is preparing a lecture on dangers of sunbathing and tanning booths for a women's group.

■ Lippincott Williams & Wilkins Multimedia Resources

Burn Care, video (1995)
Wound Care, video (1995)

■ Internet Resources

Burns: http://quickcare.org/skin/burns.html
Burns and Cancer: www.manbir-online.com/diseases/skincance.htm
Burn Emergencies: www.cl.phoenix.az.us/FIRE/burns.html

PROGRAM LICENSE AGREEMENT

Read carefully the following terms and conditions before using the Software. Use of the Software indicates you and, if applicable, your Institution's acceptance of the terms and conditions of this License Agreement. If you do not agree with the terms and conditions, you should promptly return this package to the place you purchased it and your payment will be refunded.

Definitions

As used herein, the following terms shall have the following meanings:

"Software" means the software program contained on the diskette(s) or CD-ROM or preloaded on a workstation and the user documentation, which includes all accompanying printed material.

"Institution" means a nursing or professional school, a single academic organization that does not provide patient care and is located in a single city and has one geographic location/address.

"Geographic location" means a facility at a specific location; geographic locations do not provide for satellite or remote locations that are considered a separate facility.

"Facility" means a health care facility at a specific location that provides patient care and is located in a single city and has one geographic location/address.

"Publisher" means Lippincott Williams & Wilkins, Inc., with its principal office in Philadelphia, Pennsylvania.

"Developer" means the company responsible for developing the software as noted on the product.

License

You are hereby granted a nonexclusive license to use the Software in the United States. This license is not transferable and does not authorize resale or sublicensing without the written approval or an authorized officer of Publisher. The Publisher retains all rights and title to all copyrights, patents, trademarks, trade secrets, and other proprietary rights in the Software. You may not remove or obscure the copyright notices in or on the Software. You agree to use reasonable efforts to protect the Software from unauthorized use, reproduction, distribution or publication.

Single-User license

If you purchased this Software program at the Single-User License price or a discount of that price, you may use this program on one single-user computer. You may not use the Software in a time-sharing environment or otherwise to provide multiple, simultaneous access. You may not provide or permit access to this program to anyone other than yourself.

Institutional/Facility license

If you purchased the Software at the Institutional or Facility License Price or at a discount of that price, you have purchased the Software for use within your Institution/Facility on a single workstation/computer. You may not provide copies of or remote access to the Software. You may not modify or translate the program or related documentation. You agree to instruct the individuals in your Institution/Facility who will have access to the Software to abide by the terms of this License Agreement. If you or any member of your Institution fail to comply with any of the terms of this License Agreement, this license shall terminate automatically.

Network license

If you purchased the Software at the Network License Price, you may copy the Software for use within your Institution/Facility on an unlimited number of computers within one geographic location/address. You may not provide remote access to the Software over a value-added network or otherwise. You may not provide copies of or remote access to the Software to individuals or entities who are not members of your Institution/Facility. You may not modify or translate the program or related documentation. You agree to instruct the individuals in your Institution/Facility who will have access to the Software to abide by the terms of this License Agreement. If you or any member of your Institution/Facility fail to comply with any of the terms of this License Agreement, this license shall terminate automatically.

Limited warranty

The Publisher warrants that the media on which the Software is furnished shall be free from defects in materials and workmanship under normal use for a period of 90 days from the date of delivery to you, as evidenced by your receipt of purchase.

The Software is sold on a 30-day trial basis. If, for whatever reason, you decide not to keep the software, you may return it for a full refund within 30 days of the invoice date or purchase, as evidenced by your receipt of purchase by returning all parts of the Software and packaging in saleable condition with the original invoice, to the place you purchased it. If the Software is not returned in such condition, you will not be entitled to a refund. When returning the Software, we suggest that you insure all packages for their retail value and mail them by a traceable method.

The Software is a computer assisted instruction (CAI) program that is not intended to provide medical consultation regarding the diagnosis or treatment of any specific patient.

The Software is provided without warranty of any kind, either expressed or implied, including but not limited to any implied warranty of fitness for a particular purpose of merchantability. Neither Publisher nor Developer warrants that the Software will satisfy your requirements or that the Software is free of program or content errors. Neither Publisher nor Developer warrants, guarantees, or makes any representation regarding the use of the Software in terms of accuracy, reliability or completeness, and you rely on the content of the programs solely at your own risk.

The Publisher is not responsible (as a matter of products liability, negligence or otherwise) for any injury resulting from any material contained herein. This Software contains information relating to general principles of patient care that should not be construed as specific instructions for individual patients.

Manufacturers' product information and package inserts should be reviewed for current information, including contraindications, dosages and precautions.

Some states do not allow the exclusion of implied warranties, so the above exclusion may not apply to you. This warranty gives you specific legal rights and you may also have other rights that vary from state to state.

Limitation of remedies

The entire liability of Publisher and Developer and your exclusive remedy shall be: (1) the replacement of any CD which does not meet the limited warranty stated above which is returned to the place you purchased it with your purchase receipt; or (2) if the Publisher or the wholesaler or retailer from whom you purchased the Software is unable to deliver a replacement CD free from defects in material and workmanship, you may terminate this License Agreement by returning the CD, and your money will be refunded.

In no event will Publisher or Developer be liable for any damages, including any damages for personal injury, lost profits, lost savings or other incidental or consequential damages arising out of the use or inability to use the Software or any error or defect in the Software, whether in the database or in the programming, even if the Publisher, Developer, or an authorized wholesaler or retailer has been advised of the possibility of such damage.

Some states do not allow the limitation or exclusion of liability for incidental or consequential damages. The above limitations and exclusions may not apply to you.

General

This License Agreement shall be governed by the laws of the State of Pennsylvania without reference to the conflict of laws provisions thereof, and may only be modified in a written statement signed by an authorized officer of the Publisher. By opening and using the Software, you acknowledge that you have read this License Agreement, understand it, and agree to be bound by its terms and conditions. You further agree that it is a complete and exclusive statement of the agreement between the Institution/Facility and the Publisher, which supersedes any proposal or prior agreement, oral or written, and any other communication between you and Publisher or Developer relative to the subject matter of the License Agreement.

Note

Attach a paid invoice to the License Agreement as proof of purchase.

Testbank CD-ROM to Accompany
Timby/Smith's Introductory Medical-Surgical Nursing, Eighth Edition

INSTALLATION INSTRUCTIONS

Insert the CD into the CD-ROM drive on your PC.

There are several ways to view the contents of the CD:

- Open the Start menu, go to Programs, then go to Windows Explorer. Windows Explorer will open, and you will see the icon for the CD-ROM drive on the left side of the screen. Click on the icon and the contents of the CD will appear on the right side of the screen.
- On your desktop, double-click on the "My Computer" icon. Then double-click on the icon for the CD-ROM drive. A new window will pop up with the contents of the CD.
- Hold down the Window key on your keyboard and tap the "E" key. Windows Explorer will open, and the icon for the CD-ROM drive will be on the left side of the screen. Click on the icon and the contents of the CD will appear on the right side of the screen.

Double click on any folder to view the files inside the folder.

Double click on any file to view its content.

You will need a word-processing program (e.g. MS Word or Word Perfect) to open the files on this CD.